Mariam Ghozzi
Khawla Tabbabi

What's new in the treatment of coeliac disease?

Mariam Ghozzi
Khawla Tabbabi

What's new in the treatment of coeliac disease?

gluten-free diet and new therapeutic approaches

ScienciaScripts

This book is a translation from the original published under ISBN 978-620-6-70821-6.

Publisher:
Sciencia Scripts
is a trademark of
Dodo Books Indian Ocean Ltd. and OmniScriptum S.R.L publishing group

120 High Road, East Finchley, London, N2 9ED, United Kingdom
Str. Armeneasca 28/1, office 1, Chisinau MD-2012, Republic of Moldova, Europe
Printed at: see last page
ISBN: 978-620-7-98723-8

Contents

INTRODUCTION

Celiac disease (CD) is one of the most common eating disorders in the world, affecting around 1 in 100 people worldwide [1]. It is a systemic autoimmune disease that is triggered by the ingestion of gluten, found in cereals such as wheat, rye and barley. In addition to the consumption of gluten, the development of CD is closely linked to a genetic predisposition and occurs in individuals carrying the HLA-DQ2 and/or HLA-DQ8 haplotypes. CD mainly affects the mucosa of the small intestine following the development of an immune response leading to structural changes in the intestine characterised by villous atrophy and crypt hyperplasia (elongation of the crypts) [2].

Traditionally, CD was described as a paediatric disease characterised by bloating, diarrhoea and malabsorption syndrome. However, it is now recognised as a systemic disease capable of affecting all organs and all age groups [3,4].

The clinical expression of CD is very diverse. In addition to gastrointestinal disorders, patients may present with a variety of extra-intestinal symptoms. CD may be asymptomatic. Because of this polymorphism, diagnosis remains a challenge and CD is largely under-diagnosed [2].

Diagnosis of CD is based on serological tests, duodenal histology and genetic tests. Screening aims to identify CD in subjects at risk. Screening is therefore no longer recommended for the general population [5].

In recent years, there have been major advances in our understanding of CD. However, until now, the only effective treatment available for CD has been a strict gluten-free diet (GFD). This diet must be followed for life in order to improve intestinal and extra-intestinal symptoms, regenerate intestinal villi and prevent complications of the disease. However, such a restrictive and limiting diet is generally associated with a deterioration in patients' quality of life and psychological problems. Around 40% of CD patients are dissatisfied with their diet and would like to explore alternative treatments [6]. This is why in recent years researchers have tried to respond to the growing demands of CD patients by looking for alternatives to the GFD and new therapies.

In this context, we have carried out this work with the aim of :

- Review the main characteristics and pathophysiology of CD.

- Describe the gluten-free diet and the problems associated with this treatment.

- Details of new therapeutic approaches to CD.

1. GENERAL INFORMATION ABOUT COELIAC DISEASE

1.1 Definition

The word 'coeliac' literally comes from the Greek 'koliakos' meaning 'suffering of the intestine' [7].

CD is a chronic autoimmune inflammatory enteropathy secondary to the ingestion of gliadin from wheat, and related prolamins from barley and rye, occurring in genetically predisposed individuals with the HLA-DQ2 and/or HLA-DQ8 phenotype. It is manifested by the presence of serological markers and histological flattening of the intestinal villi **(Figure 1) [8]**. Some CD patients may also be affected by avenin (the protein found in oats) [9].

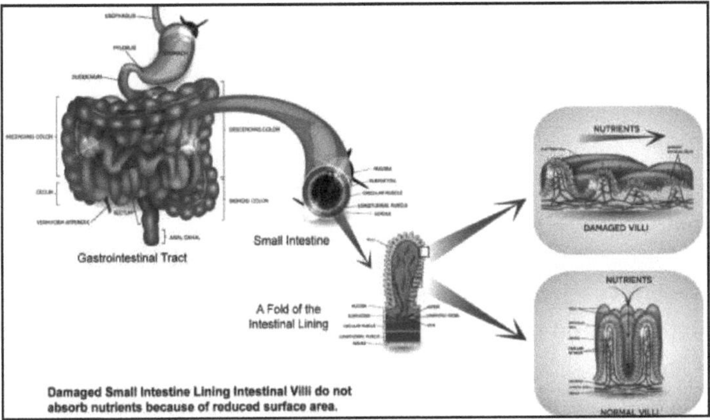

Figure 1: Difference between atrophied intestinal villi in the course of

celiac disease and normal intestinal villi [10].

Understanding the pathophysiological phenomena involving the adaptive immune response and the innate immune response has enabled a clear distinction to be made between CD and gluten allergy [11].

1.2 Epidemiology

CD is one of the most common autoimmune diseases, with a prevalence in the general population of between 0.5 and 1% [6]. Prevalence in Europe varies from 0.3% in Germany to 2% in Finland. In North Africa, prevalence is 0.79% in Libya, 0.53% in Egypt and 0.6% in Tunisia. In Saudi Arabia, it ranges from 2.1% to 8.5% [12]. In contrast, CD remains virtually exceptional in South-East Asia, in China (0.1%-0.5%) and Japan (<0.1%), and in sub-Saharan Africa [13,14]. Taking into account the various clinical expressions of CD (gastrointestinal signs, extraintestinal signs or absence of symptoms), the actual prevalence of CD has increased over the last 30 years and up to 83% of patients with this disease are not diagnosed according to a study carried out in the United States [15,16]. An epidemiological study published in 2007, carried out in a school environment in the Ariana governorate and involving 6,284 Tunisian schoolchildren, used IgA anti-transglutaminase (TG) 2 antibodies as a screening method. The results showed a prevalence of CD of 1/157, with the majority of children screened presenting atypical or silent forms [17]. CD affects women 2 to 3 times more than men [12]. It can affect all age groups. However, the incidence is approximately 2 times higher in children than in adults, with an incidence of 21.3/100,000 people per year compared with 12.9 in adults [18].

Several studies have identified a risk group encompassing subjects who are more likely to develop CD and who are those having [19]:

- A first-degree relative (parents, siblings) with CD.
- Another autoimmune disease, in particular type I diabetes and Hashimoto's thyroiditis.
- IgA deficiency.
- A genetic anomaly such as trisomy 21, Turner syndrome or Williams-Beuren syndrome.

1.3 Etiopathogenesis

CD is a multifactorial disease. Its onset depends on genetic predisposition and the intervention of environmental factors.

1.3.1. Environmental factors

1.3.1.1. Gluten

Gluten is a group of proteins that are essential for dough formation because of their unique viscoelastic properties [2]. These proteins are classified into two families with different solubilities in alcohol: prolamins and glutelins. The prolamins in wheat, rye and barley are known to be toxic to people with CD. In each species of these three cereals, this fraction is designated by specific names: gliadin for wheat, hordenin for barley and secalin for rye. Gliadins, which are the toxic prolamins of wheat, are monomeric proteins classified according to their electrophoretic mobility into four groups: α-, β-, γ-, ω- gliadins [20].

The toxicity of prolamins is mainly due to their high proline content, which makes them resistant to enzymatic degradation and is responsible for the high immunogenicity of gluten. In fact, a high proportion (80%) of this amino acid prevents complete proteolysis of gluten by the enzymes of the brush border of the intestine and the gastric and pancreatic enzymes, leaving very long peptides which reach the mucosa of the small intestine and are responsible for the inflammation and autoimmune response in gluten-intolerant subjects [9].

1.3.1.2. Alteration of the intestinal microbiota

Alterations in the microbiota contribute to many chronic immune disorders, such as CD. Several mechanisms have been proposed to elucidate the involvement of the gut microbiota in the pathogenesis of CD and loss of gluten tolerance. In recent years, numerous studies have examined the faecal, salivary and duodenal microbiota in coeliac patients. A decrease in beneficial species, such as *Lactobacillus* and *Bifidobacterium*, and an increase in pathogenic species, such as *Bacteroides* and *Escherichia coli*, compared with healthy subjects have been observed. *Lactobacilli* and *Bifidobacterium* contribute to the degradation of gluten, leading to changes in its immunogenic potential. Studies have shown that opportunistic pathogens and intestinal commensals have distinct gluten degradation patterns, leading to increased or decreased immunogenicity, which may influence the risk of autoimmunity. Moreover, *Lactobacillus* are capable of detoxifying immunogenic peptides after they have been partially digested by human proteases. What's more, in the presence of *Lactobacillus*, the immunogenic peptides produced by *P.aeruginosa* proteases are also degraded, making them less immunogenic **(Figure 2)**. Other research has demonstrated a relationship between dysbiosis and an increase in the release of zonulin, which disrupts the integrity of tight junctions and promotes the penetration of partially digested gliadin peptides into the lamina propria **[21,22]**.

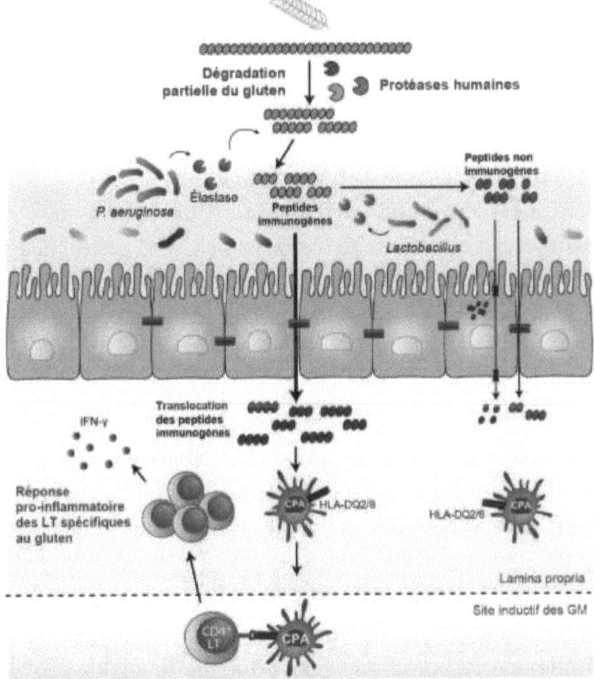

APC: antigen-presenting cell; TL: T lymphocytes; GM: mesenteric lymph nodes; HLA: *Human Leukocyte Antigen*; IFN: interferon; CD: *Cluster of differentiation*;

Figure 2: Modulation of the pathogenesis of coeliac disease during gluten digestion in the presence of *P. aeruginosa* and *Lactobacillus* [23].

1.3.1.3. Age of introduction of gluten and breastfeeding

Numerous studies have been carried out to assess the role of the age of introduction of gluten and breastfeeding in the prevention of CD. The results of these studies are contradictory. According to the latest 2016 recommendations of the *European Society for Paediatric Gastroenterology Hepatology and Nutrition* (ESPGHAN), gluten should be introduced into the diet between the fourth and twelfth months [24]. Consumption of large quantities of gluten is not recommended during the first few months following the introduction of gluten to breastfed infants. In fact, breastfeeding offers protection against CD due to the presence of immunocompetent factors that strengthen the child's immune system against gastrointestinal infections. In addition, breast milk stimulates the maturation of the immune system of the intestinal mucosa, as it contains a large quantity of microRNA. These small non-coding RNA molecules regulate at the post-transcriptional level the expression of genes involved in the mechanisms of cell proliferation and apoptosis [25]. However, the *European Society for the Study of Coeliac Disease* (ESsCD) published in 2019 in the European Journal of Gastroenterology that the duration of breastfeeding and the time of introduction of gluten have no impact on the risk of developing CD. To date, there is no recommendation regarding the early (at 4 months) or late (at 6 or even 12 months) introduction of gluten in at-risk children [8].

1.3.1.4 Viral and bacterial intestinal infections

Intestinal infections can contribute to the onset of CD in genetically predisposed individuals in a variety of ways. Repeated viral infections in childhood may affect the maturation of the intestinal defence system and predispose the child to further bacterial infections and long-term changes in the gut microbiota [26]. A recent study [27] revealed that children exposed to *enteroviruses* before the age of three had a higher risk of developing CD later in life. This is because *enteroviruses* provoke an excessive immune response in the gut, leading to disruption of the intestinal mucosal barrier, which results in increased translocation of gluten peptides into the mucosa and increased intestinal permeability. In addition, *enteroviruses* emit a danger signal, activating dendritic cells that present the TG2-modified gluten peptides to gluten-reactive *cluster of differentiation* (CD) 4 T lymphocytes (LT), which are responsible for the abnormal immune response and hence for the breakdown of tolerance to gluten peptides.

In addition, *reovirus* infection leads to increased type 1 interferon (INF) signalling and increased expression of INF regulatory transcription factor 1, which blocks the conversion of LTs into regulatory CD4 LTs and thus promotes a pro-inflammatory response to food antigens [4].

Various studies have also shown that infections, mainly those induced by *Clostridium difficile* and *Helicobacter pylori,* can play a role in inducing CD. The incidence of *Clostridium difficile* infection in a group of CD patients has been estimated at 56/100,000 people per year. In addition, almost 63% of patients with CD have *Helicobacter pylori* infection [28]. A recent study showed that duodenal biopsies from patients with CD showed elevated proteolytic activity correlated with the proliferation of specific opportunistic pathogens such as *Pseudomonas.* The onset of the disease has been linked to an increase in intestinal permeability by various mechanisms such as the activation of receptors (*"Toll like receptors"* (TLR) or *"Protease activated receptors"* (PAR)) leading to the production of pro-inflammatory cytokines or the modification of the components of the intestinal barrier (tight junctions or intestinal mucosa) leading to a breakdown in gluten tolerance [26].

1.3.2. Genetic predisposition

A genetic predisposition in patients with CD has been demonstrated by concordance studies in monozygotic twins (75%-80%) and studies of the transmission of the disease in first-degree relatives (~10%-15%   )   [13]. Genetic factors in CD particularly involve the HLA (*"Human Leukocyte Antigen"*) system, which is encoded by the HLA genes located on chromosome 6 (6p21), comprising three sub-regions: HLA-DP, HLA-DQ and HLA-DR [29]. Approximately 95% of CD patients express the DQ2 molecule and the remaining 5% of patients express the DQ8 molecule [1]. The HLA-DQ molecule is a heterodimer composed of an alpha chain encoded by the HLA-DQA1 gene and a beta chain encoded by the HLA- DQB1 gene. The two components of this heterodimer are encoded by the HLA- DQA1 and HLA-DQB1 genes in cis (inherited by the same parent) or in trans (inherited by each of the two parents) **(Figure 3) [30]**.

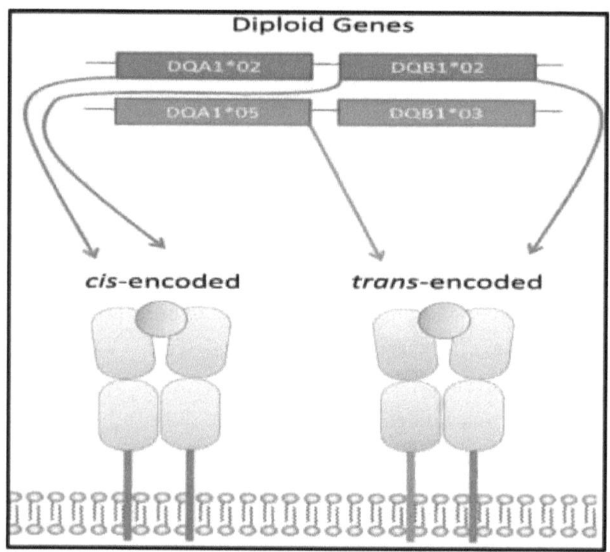

Figure 3: Representation of a *cis*- and *trans*-encoded HLA-DQ molecule [30].

The different HLA-DQ serotypes are essentially derived from polymorphism of the DQA1 and DQB1 chains. For each serotype, there are several alleles corresponding to it **(Table I)**. The HLA-DQB1*02 allele of HLA- DQ2.5 and HLA-DQ2.2 confer a higher risk of CD than the HLA-DQB1*03 allele of HLA-DQ8 **[5,31]**.

Table I: Correspondence between the serotype and the alleles responsible for

celiac disease [30].

Alleles HLA-DQAI	Alleles HLA-DQBI	Haplotype	Serotype
DQA1*05	DQB1*02	DQ2.5	DQ2
DQA1*03	DQB1*03	DQ8	DQ8
DQA1*02	DQB1*02	DQ2.2	DQ2

HLA: *Human Leukocyte Antigen*

The presence of an HLA-DQ2 and/or DQ8 haplotype is the main risk factor for CD. These haplotypes are present in almost 30% of the general population, whereas only around 1% of the population has CD, demonstrating that their presence is essential but not sufficient to develop the disease **[30]**.

1.4 Pathophysiology of coeliac disease
1.4.1. Degradation of gluten

In the intestinal lumen, gluten is broken down by digestive enzymes, releasing peptide sequences containing a toxic (immunogenic) fragment. Due to the absence of a prolyl-endopeptidase activity capable of cleaving peptides containing prolin residues, these peptide sequences are resistant to gastrointestinal proteases and to the enzymes of the brush border membrane of the small intestine. This resistance of immunogenic peptides is due to their unique amino acid composition, with a high proline (15%) and glutamine (35%) content and a high percentage of hydrophobic amino acids (19%). The immunogenic peptides resulting from this incomplete digestion will induce innate and adaptive immune responses [32,33].

1.4.2. Crossing the epithelial barrier

An alteration in intestinal permeability is observed in individuals with CD. At the level of the epithelial wall, the binding of gliadin to CXCR3 membrane receptors triggers the secretion of zonulin, which is considered to be a modulator of intestinal tight junctions [34,35]. The secretion of zonulin by enterocytes induces an alteration in intercellular tight junction proteins, leading to their relaxation. The result is an increase in intestinal permeability, which favours the paracellular passage of gliadin towards the subepithelial compartment **(Figure 4)** [34,36].

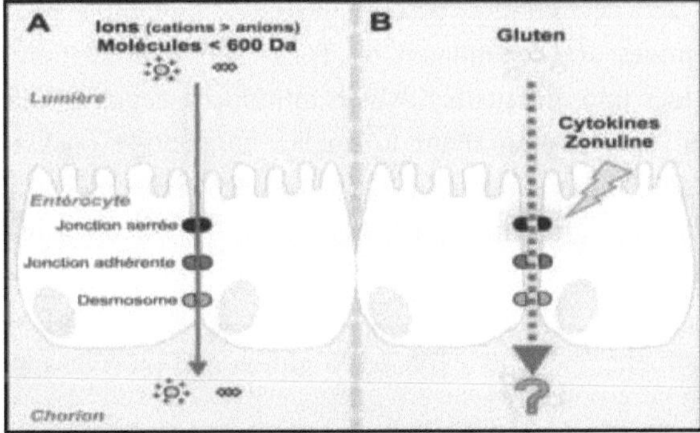

Figure 4: Paracellular transport of gluten under physiological conditions and in coeliac disease [34].

The mechanism of gliadin transport via the transcellular pathway is closely linked to the CD71 receptor. Under physiological conditions, CD71 is found exclusively in the basement membrane of enterocytes located in the crypts. In a coeliac patient, CD71 is over-expressed in the epithelium of the apical membrane of the enterocytes. This overexpression may be due to various causes, such as iron deficiency, inflammation or infection **(Figure 5) [34]**.

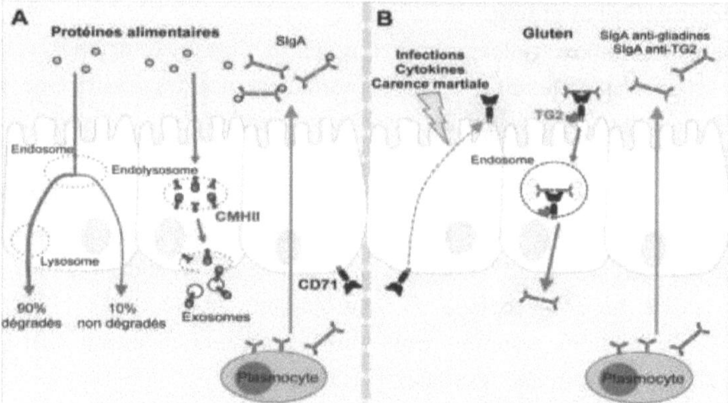

MHC: Histocompatibility Complex; CD: *Cluster of differentiation*; SIgA:
Secretory immunoglobulin A; TG2: Transglutaminase 2

Figure 5   **Transcellular transport of gluten under
physiological conditions
(A) and in celiac disease (B) [34].**

5.4.3. Formation of a gliadin-transglutaminase 2 complex in the lamina propria

TG2 is a ubiquitous multifunctional enzyme. It catalyses two types of reaction: transamidation and deamidation of the substrate's glutamine residues. During CD, gluten peptides are deamidated by TG2. This deamidation converts the glutamine residues into glutamates, which introduces negative charges into the gluten peptides, encouraging them to anchor in peptide pockets formed by positively charged amino acids (HLA-DQ2 or DQ8 molecules), thus forming a complex which is recognised by LTs **(Figure 6)**. On the other hand, the TG2-desamide peptide complex of gliadin acts as an autoantigen which stimulates the production of specific IgA, which explains the appearance of autoantibodies against TG2 in coeliac patients exposed to gluten and their disappearance after GFD **[37]**.

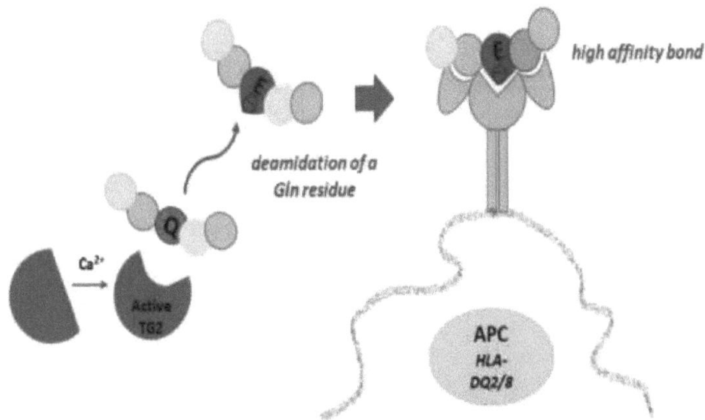

HLA: *Human leucocyte antigen system;* Ca^2 +: Calcium cation; APC: *Antigen presenting cell*; TG2: Transglutaminase 2; Gln: gliadin

Figure 6   Deamidation of a gliadin peptide by transglutaminase 2 and recognition by DQ2/8 molecules located on antigen-presenting cells antigen-presenting cells [37].

6.4.4. Role of innate immunity

The pathophysiology of CD involves an innate immune response which constitutes the body's first line of defence. It involves different types of cells and molecular players that play an important role in antigen presentation and the production of cytokines that amplify the adaptive immune response. IL-15 and -18 play a major role in innate immunity by inducing the proliferation and recruitment of intraepithelial lymphocytes (IELs) in the intestinal mucosa, and by promoting their cytotoxic action through the expression of molecules such as Fas ligand (FasL), perforin, granzyme B and *natural killer group 2 member D* (NKG2D) [2]. The α-gliadin peptide 31-43 is able to penetrate epithelial cells, triggering an innate immune response and activating the epithelial stress process. This activation leads to overexpression of IL-15 by enterocytes and mononuclear cells in the lamina propria. Overexpression of IL-15 stimulates expression of MICA/B (stress molecules and NKG2D receptor ligand) in enterocytes and expression of *natural killer* (NK) cell receptors, inducing a cytotoxic response against epithelial cells **(Figure 7) [38].** In addition, peptide 31-43 can activate the *Mitogen-activated protein* (MAP) kinase signalling pathway. This pathway is involved in the regulation of enterocyte growth, differentiation and survival, promoting epithelial cell proliferation and contributing to intestinal crypt hyperplasia **[39].** In CD, high levels of pro-inflammatory cytokines such as IFN-γ and IL-15 have been detected in intestinal lesions. These cytokines contribute to disease progression by promoting inflammation and disrupting the anti-inflammatory immune response. IL-15, as a pleiotropic cytokine, promotes inflammation in a number of ways. It induces the accumulation of cytotoxic intra-epithelial lymphocytes in the mucosal lesions observed in coeliac patients. It also disrupts the suppressive activity of regulatory LT and interferes with *Transforming Growth Factor* (TGF) β signalling. It also activates CD4+ T lymphocytes. In addition, IL-15 can lead to the development of T lymphoma through the expansion of aberrant ILL clones [4].

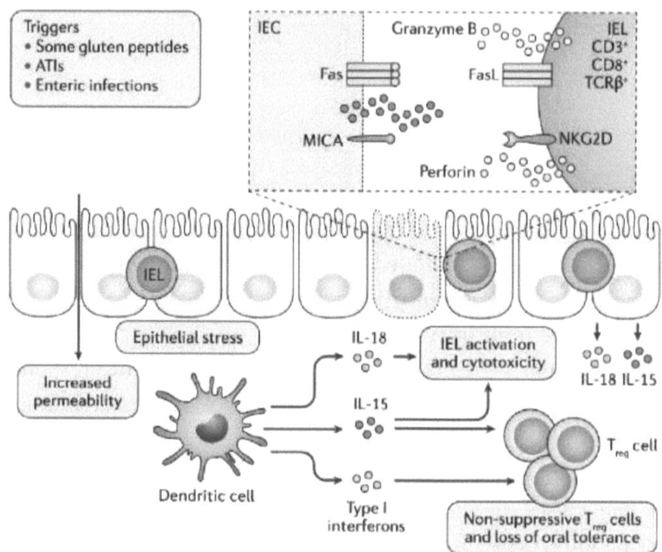

ATI: *"α- Amylase-Trypsin inhibitors"*; IL: Interleukin; IEL: *"Intraepithelial lymphocytes"*; IEC: *"Intestinal epithelial cells"*; FasL: Fas ligand; NKG2D: *"Natural Killer group 2 member D"*; MICA: *"Major histocompatibility complex class I chain- related protein A"*; Treg: T regulatory lymphocyte; TCRβ: *"T-cell receptor beta"*; CD: *Cluster of differentiation*

Figure 7   Innate immune response involved in coeliac disease [2].

7.4.5. Role of adaptive immunity

In the lamina propria, the gluten peptide transported and deamidated by TG2 will bind to HLA-DQ2 or DQ-8 molecules expressed on the surface of antigen-presenting cells (APCs), inducing activation of intestinal CD4+ LTs and activating a cascade of inflammatory reactions. Activation of CD4+ LTs leads to the release of pro-inflammatory cytokines such as IFN-γ and *Tumor necrosis factor* (TNF) α. These cytokines stimulate *T-helper* (TH) 1 lymphocytes to produce IL-15 and IL-21, leading to the activation of cytotoxic CD8+ ILLs,

which cause intestinal lesions **(figure 8).**
[40].

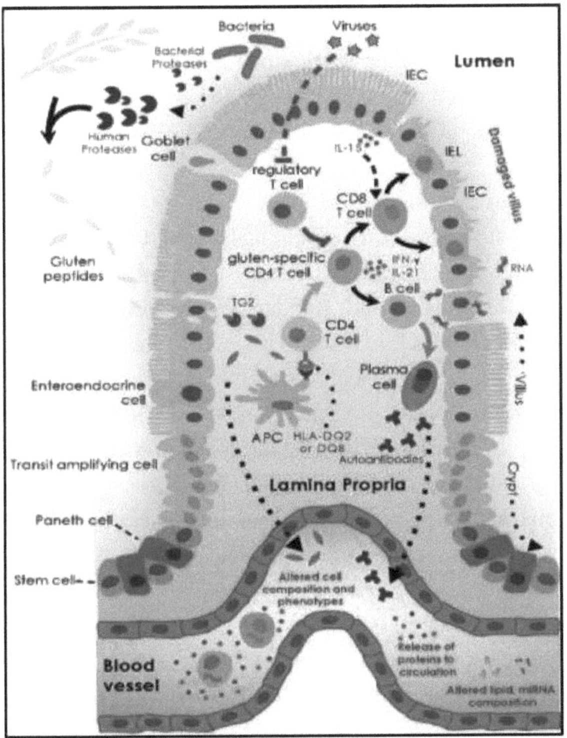

APC: *Antigen presenting cell*; TG2: Transglutaminase 2; CD: *Cluster of differentiation*; T
cell: T lymphocyte; B cell: B lymphocyte; IFN: Interferon; IL:
Interleukin; HLA: *Human leukocyte antigen system*; IEC: *Intraepithelial
lymphocytes"*; IEL: *"Intestinal epithelial cells"*; RNA: *"Ribonucleic acid"*;

Figure 8   Immune responses involved in celiac disease [41].
In addition, B lymphocytes (LB) undergo differentiation into plasma cells
secreting anti-gliadin Ac (AAG), anti-gliadin desamide peptide (PGD) Ac, anti-
endomysium Ac (AAE), and anti-TG2 Ac under the effect of TH2 lymphocytes.
Antibodies, particularly anti-gliadin IgG and anti-TG2 IgA, promote activation
of the classical complement pathway, leading to increased production of C3a
and C5a. These anaphylatoxins increase vascular permeability and trigger
degranulation of the mast cells responsible for lesions and villous atrophy. Anti-
TG2 antibodies may also play a role in enterocyte differentiation by blocking
TGF-β activation. Anti-TG2 antibodies bind to TG2 and disrupt its interaction
with TGF-β. This will prevent the activation of this cytokine and potentially
affect enterocyte differentiation **[42]**. An analysis of non-gluten-stimulated

CD4+ T cells from the blood of CD patients showed a significant increase in IFN-γ gene expression and a decrease in BACH2 gene expression. The combination of these two factors leads to an inflammatory state mediated by TH1 lymphocytes. On the other hand, since BACH2 is an immune regulatory transcription factor, a reduction in its expression will lead to an increase in effector TLs and a decrease in regulatory TLs, which also promotes inflammation [4].

1.5. Clinical forms of coeliac disease

CD is a real chameleon in terms of clinical form. It can present in different forms [43]. In 2011, the Oslo classification was used to describe the different clinical presentations of CD and standardise the nomenclature used in the scientific and clinical literature [44]. However, since its publication, some experts have criticised the "classical / non-classical" categorisation for not fully reflecting the current clinical presentations of CD [6]. "In 2016, the *World Gastroenterology Organisation Global Guidelines Celiac Disease* proposed an alternative classification of CD based on the 2011 Oslo classification. In 2020, ESPGHAN published a description based on the presence or absence of clinical symptoms, as well as the results of serological tests and small bowel biopsies [45].

1.5.1. Symptomatic forms

1.5.1.1. Classic symptomatic form

In this classic form, diarrhoea with profuse stools is the most frequent manifestation of CD in children. It may be accompanied by nausea, anorexia and apathy. Recurrent vomiting, delayed growth or puberty and short stature are also characteristic of classic CD [43]. In adults, diarrhoea remains a major symptom associated with bloating, abdominal pain and weight loss [6].

1.5.1.2. Non-classical symptomatic form

In recent years, the non-classical symptomatic form, in which digestive symptoms are less pronounced or absent, has become increasingly common. It is most often manifested by extradigestive signs. The most suggestive signs may include anaemia, osteoporosis, dermatitis herpetiformis and neurological disorders [6,43].

1.5.2. Asymptomatic form

CD can also present in an asymptomatic form. Because of this insidious clinical presentation, CD is often discovered by chance. In fact, the patient presents no suggestive clinical signs despite positive serological tests (presence of serum antibodies) and the presence of characteristic histological lesions on duodenal biopsy [6,46].

1.5.3. Potential form

According to the latest ESPGHAN recommendations of 2020, the potential form of CD is characterised by the presence of high levels of anti-TG2 Ac and anti-endomysial Ac (EAA) in the blood with no histological lesions or only minor changes. People with this form may be asymptomatic or may present with classic or atypical symptoms of CD [3,45].

1.5.4. Latent form

There is often confusion between the terms "latent form" and "potential form" of CD. For this reason, experts have decided to avoid using the term "latent" to describe this form of CD, opting instead for the term "potential" [44].

1.5.5. Refractory form

The refractory form of CD is characterised by the presence of clinical symptoms and a malabsorption syndrome that persist or recur, with the presence of villous atrophy despite strict GFD for more than 12 months. Refractory CD is classified into two types according to the percentage of aberrant LIE expression [46] :

- Type I: the proportion of aberrant LELs is less than 20%.
- Type II: the proportion of aberrant LELs is greater than 20%. This form is considered to be pre-lymphoma or low-grade lymphoma.

1.5.6. Seronegative form

Seronegative CD is a form of CD that is not described by the Oslo classification. According to the American Gastrological Association's 2021 recommendations, this form is defined by the presence of an active histological abnormality accompanied by negative serology for anti-TG2 Ac, anti PDG Ac and AAE and compatible genetics in patients with or without gastrointestinal signs and symptoms, excluding any other cause of enteropathy [47].

1.6.Clinical manifestations

Although CD is defined as an enteropathy, its symptomatic expression is extremely variable, including gastrointestinal symptoms and extra-intestinal manifestations **(Figure 9) [3].**

Dental enamel hypoplasia Recurrent aphthous mouth ulceration

Figure 9: Clinical manifestations of coeliac disease [2].

1.6.1. Digestive disorders

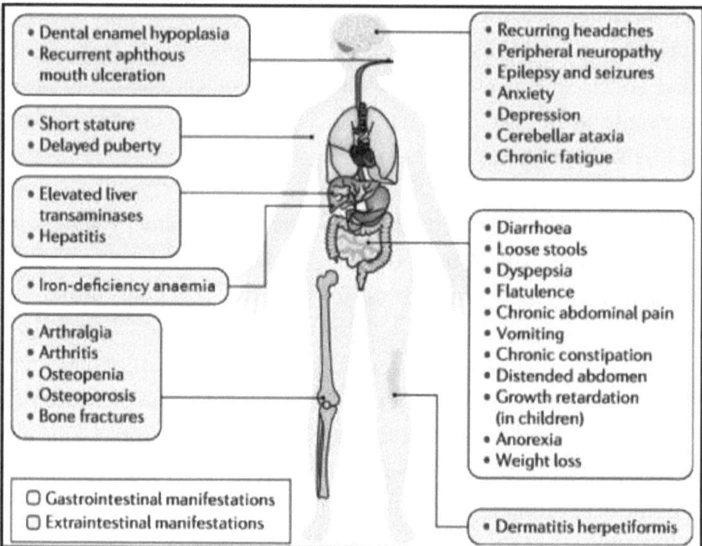

The gastrointestinal presentation of CD is characterised by a range of clinical signs of varying intensity. In children under the age of 3, symptoms may include diarrhoea, loss of appetite and abdominal distension. Older children and adults may also present with these symptoms, as well as constipation, bloating, abdominal pain and weight loss. On the other hand, a clinical picture combining chronic diarrhoea with malabsorption syndrome, weight loss and significant asthenia is fairly rare in adults. In rare cases, serious consequences may be observed, such as cachexia, sarcopenia, significant hypoalbuminemia and electrolyte imbalance requiring hospitalisation. However, a presentation similar to irritable bowel syndrome is quite common. This is manifested by constipation or alternating diarrhoea and constipation and/or dyspepsia-like symptoms, such as nausea and sometimes vomiting [6].

1.6.2. Extradigestive manifestations

According to the latest studies, extradigestive manifestations tend to be the most frequent in children and adults **(Figure 9)** [6].

1.6.2.1.   Osteoarticular manifestations

Osteoporosis is the most common osteoarticular manifestation of CD, affecting up to 70% of patients. The damage caused to the intestinal mucosa by gluten ingestion reduces the absorption of calcium and vitamin D, two nutrients essential for maintaining bone density, and increases the risk of bone fractures. In children, stunted growth and short stature may indicate CD [2,5]. Osteomalacia characterised by muscle weakness, bone pain and spontaneous fractures secondary to reduced vitamin D absorption may also be observed in coeliac patients. Arthralgia and arthritis are also common in CD patients. Approximately 20-30% of patients report joint pain at the time of diagnosis of CD [48].

1.6.2.2.   Haematological manifestations

Iron deficiency anaemia is the second most common presentation of CD. CD exposes patients to martial deficiency due to malabsorption of iron. It results in a microcytic anaemia observed in around 40% of cases [49]. More rarely, coeliac patients may suffer from vitamin B12 and folate deficiency, which leads to macrocytic anaemia. Leukopenia and thrombocytopenia may also be observed [6]. Coagulation abnormalities associated with defective vitamin K absorption have been described in some cases of CD [50].

1.6.2.3.   Neurological manifestations

The relationship between CD and neurological disorders was first described in 1966 by Dr Cooke and Dr Smith, who observed signs of cerebellar ataxia and peripheral neuropathy in patients with CD. Cerebellar ataxia, known as gluten ataxia, is often one of the first neurological symptoms to appear. Coeliac patients affected by gluten ataxia have a particular type of neurological deficit, which is the loss of Purkinje cells. Initially, this damage was attributed to vitamin deficiencies in vitamins B1, B3, B6 or B12. However, recent studies have shown that AAGs and anti-TG2 antibodies have an affinity for the deep cerebellar nuclei, brainstem neurons and cortex, leading to cross-reactivity with common epitopes in Purkinje cells and thus causing their damage. The second most common neurological manifestation reported in CD patients is peripheral neuropathy. This is often discovered as a result of difficulty writing, a tingling sensation and reduced sensitivity to pain or heat on contact with the skin [51]. Other neurological manifestations associated with CD include headache and epilepsy. Around 20% of coeliac patients suffer from headaches. In children with CD, the prevalence of epilepsy is 1.5 times higher than in the general population [3].

1.6.2.4.   Impact of coeliac disease on fertility

CD is considered to be a risk factor for infertility. Clinical and epidemiological data have shown that CD affects the male and female reproductive systems. CD can be associated with delayed puberty, early menopause, amenorrhoea and reduced fertility. Several studies have shown that CD can increase the risk of miscarriage and premature birth in pregnant coeliac patients [3,6]. In the male population suffering from CD, abnormalities in sperm morphology and motility may be observed [51].

1.6.2.5. Mucocutaneous manifestations

There is evidence that CD patients are at risk of developing a variety of skin disorders, such as dermatitis herpetiformis, psoriasis, atopic dermatitis, urticaria and patchy alopecia. Dermatitis herpetiformis is the most common dermatological manifestation of CD [48,51]. Around 10% of adults with coeliac disease develop dermatitis herpetiformis, characterised by pruritic papulovesicular lesions, particularly on the elbows, knees, buttocks and scalp [2].

1.7. Diagnosis of coeliac disease

1.7.1. Clinical diagnosis

The onset of clinical symptoms is one of the key factors in the diagnosis of CD. For this reason, the clinical examination must be meticulous if the diagnosis of CD is not to be missed [46].

1.7.2. Serological diagnosis

Over the last 20 years, the use of serological tests has led to a significant increase in diagnosed cases of CD. The serological markers of CD are classified into two groups [6]:

- Autoantibodies targeting autoantigens: AAE and anti-TG2 antibodies
- Acids targeting toxic prolamins: AAG and anti-PGD Acids

The antibodies observed in CD are of the IgA and IgG isotypes. Only IgA antibodies are considered to be highly specific for CD. However, IgG antibodies are sought in patients with IgA deficiency [6].

1.7.2.1. Anti-gliadin antibodies

The anti-gliadin antibody was the first serological marker for CD to be developed in the early 1980s. At the time, it was widely used to diagnose CD. However, due to its lack of sensitivity and specificity, this serological test is no longer recommended for screening patients at risk of CD and has been replaced by more sensitive and specific serological tests. Its role is now limited to identifying subjects with non-celiac intolerance to gluten [6,8].

1.7.2.2. Anti-endomysial antibodies and anti-transglutaminase 2 antibodies

Testing for EAA and IgA anti-TG2 isotype antibodies is the gold standard for the biological diagnosis of CD. These two tests have a sensitivity and specificity of over 95%. IgA-isotype EAAs are tested by indirect immunofluorescence (IFI) on sections of monkey oesophagus **(figure 10)** or on sections of human umbilical cord. IgA anti-TG2 autoantibodies, on the other hand, are detected by *enzyme-linked immunosorbent assay* (ELISA). These two autoantibodies are often presented as equivalent, since they are directed against the same autoantigen: TG2. In fact, the test for anti-TG2 IgA isotype antibodies is more sensitive than that for IgA isotype AAEs, but it is less specific. The latter is more expensive and requires an experienced observer to interpret the IFI results correctly. It is used as a confirmatory test, particularly when the anti-TG2 titre is less than 2 times the positivity threshold [8,52].

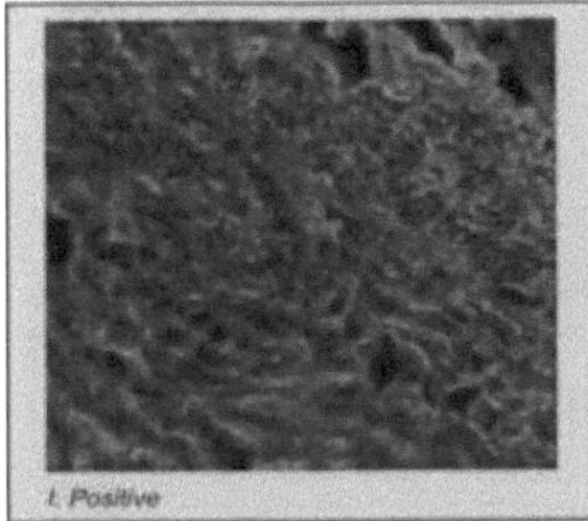

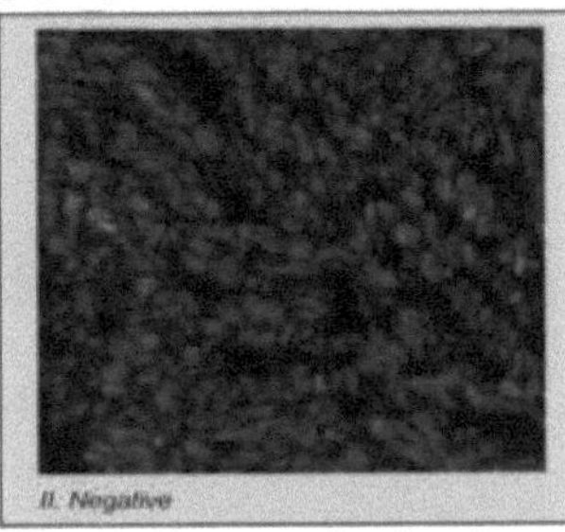

I) Presence of anti-endomysial IgA antibodies, II) Absence of anti-endomysial IgA antibodies.

Figure 10: Indirect immunofluorescence performed on a section of monkey oesophagus [53].

1.7.2.3. Antibodies to deamidated peptides of gliadin

IgG or IgA anti-PDG antibodies are tested by ELISA and have no advantage over anti-TG2 antibodies. Testing for anti-PDG IgG is the test of choice for patients with IgA deficiency or for children under the age of two, since the sensitivity of other tests is low before this age [8,54].

1.7.3. Histological diagnosis and endoscopy

1.7.3.1. Endoscopy

Despite the limited sensitivity and specificity for detecting CD, certain endoscopic findings should raise doubts and arouse suspicion. These duodenal findings include **(Figure 11)**:

- Fold irregularity
- Fissuring of the folds and a mosaic-like appearance of the mucosa
- Flattening of folds and/or disappearance of folds
- Reduction in the number and size of folds
- Absence of villi at high magnification
- Granular appearance of the bulbar part of the duodenum

Approximately one-third of newly diagnosed coeliac patients have a normal endoscopic appearance. Therefore, when CD is suspected, biopsies should be performed even in the presence of a normal endoscopic appearance [8,55].

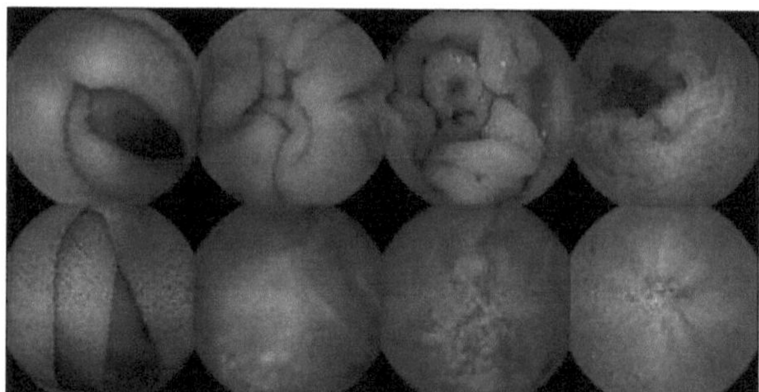

Figure 11: Endoscopic image of the mucosa of the small intestine [56] top row: healthy individual, bottom row: coeliac patient

1.7.3.2. Duodenal biopsies

For a long time, duodenal biopsies were considered the *"gold standard"* for diagnosing CD. Due to the irregular distribution of CD lesions, it is recommended that several samples be taken from different sites [46] :

- Four biopsies from the second part of the duodenum
- Two others in the duodenal bulb.

Several classifications have been proposed to determine the severity of villous atrophy. Currently, the Marsh classification modified by Oberhüber **(Table II)** is the most widely used by pathologists for the initial diagnosis and to assess the regression of lesions caused by CD after RSG [8].

Table II: Marsh-Oberhüber classification [57].

Histological criteria			
Type	LEL > 25 per 100 epithelial cells	Crypt hyperplasia	Villi atrophy
Type 1	Yes	No	No
Type 2	Yes	Yes	No
Type 3a	Yes	Yes	Partial
Type 3b	Yes	Yes	Subtotal
Type 3c	Yes	Yes	Total

IEL: Intraepithelial lymphocytes

Corazza and Villanacc proposed a simpler grading system **(Table III)** to facilitate comparison between follow-up biopsies [8].

Table III: Corazza and Villanacci classification [57].

Histological criteria			
Grade	LEL > 25 per 100 epithelial cells	Crypt hyperplasia	Villi atrophy

Grade A	Yes	No	No
Grade B1	Yes	Yes	Partial
Grade B2	Yes	Yes	Total

IEL: Intraepithelial lymphocytes

1.7.4. HLA typing

The presence of the HLA-DQ2 and HLA-DQ8 molecules is an essential genetic risk factor for developing CD. HLA typing is not routinely performed to diagnose CD, given that 30% to 40% of the general population carry the HLA-DQ2 and/or HLA-DQ8 genes [46]. When the HLA-DQ2/8 test is negative, the diagnosis of CD is highly unlikely (positive predictive value greater than 99%). HLA genotyping is recommended in the following situations [8]:

• Presence of characteristic histological damage with negative serology, or vice versa.

• Identification of subjects at risk who have a first-degree relative (parents, siblings) with CD so that screening can be considered.

• Patients with other autoimmune diseases and/or genetic disorders at risk of developing CD.

1.7.5. New recommendations

1.7.5.1.   For children

The diagnosis of CD in children can be challenging due to the diversity of clinical manifestations and the difficulty in identifying specific symptoms in this population **(Figure 12)**. Many children with CD present with atypical or asymptomatic forms of the disease, where classic digestive symptoms may be absent or masked by other clinical manifestations, making diagnosis particularly complex **(Figure 13) [58]**.

IgA: Immunoglobulin A; TG2: Transglutaminase 2; 10N: 10 times normal; EM: Endomysium; EDH: Upper gastrointestinal endoscopy;

DGP: *Deamidated gliadin peptide*

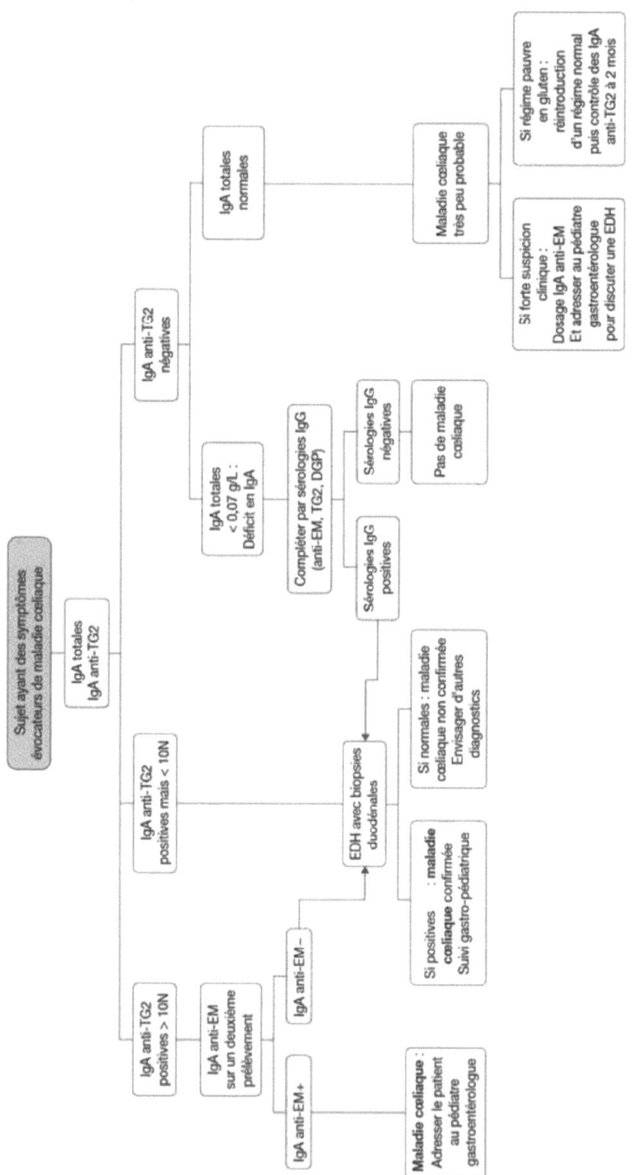

Figure 12: Diagnostic algorithm for coeliac disease in the symptomatic paediatric population [58].

22

IgA: immunoglobulin A; TG2: transglutaminase 2; 10N: 10 times normal; EM: endomysium; EDH: upper digestive endoscopy; DGP: "Deamidated gliadin peptide; HLA: Human leucocyte antigen system.

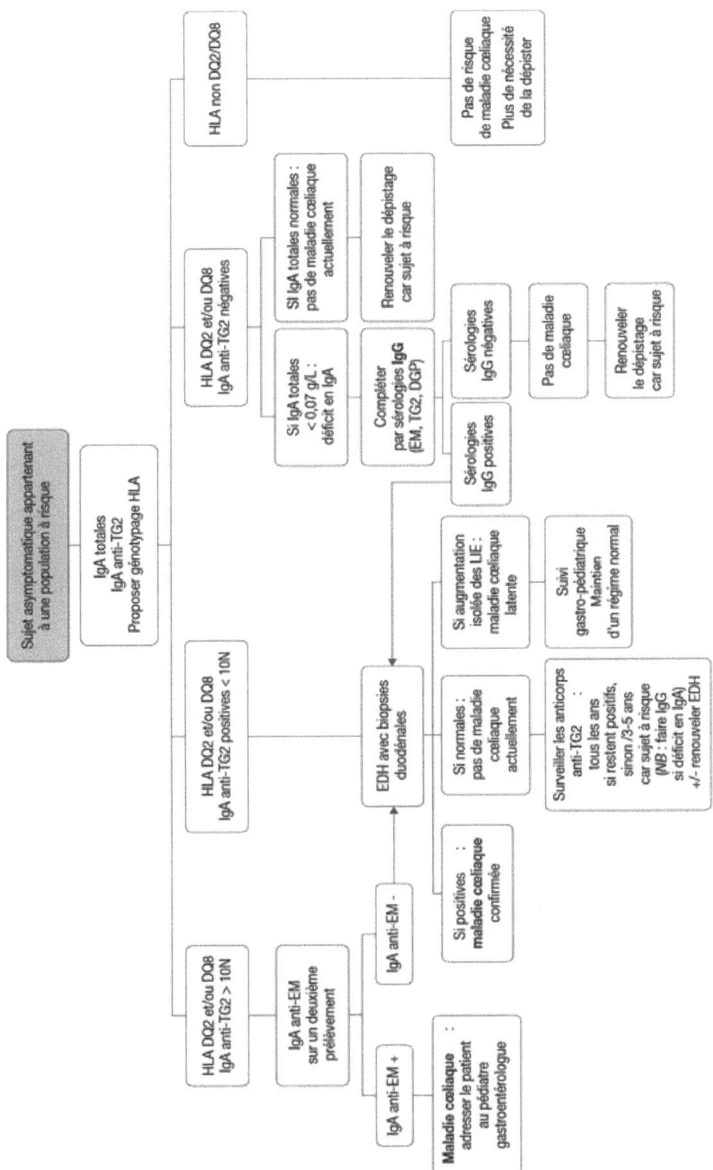

Figure 13: Diagnosis of coeliac disease in asymptomatic children at risk [58].

In adults, it is recommended to begin by measuring total IgA, followed by anti-TG2 IgA. Then, depending on the level of anti-TG2 IgA, duodenal biopsies or other serological tests (IgA AAE, anti-TG2 IgG, anti-PDG IgG) should be performed **(Figure 14) [6]**. HLA typing is not recommended for the initial diagnosis of CD, but it may help to exclude the disease **[8]**.

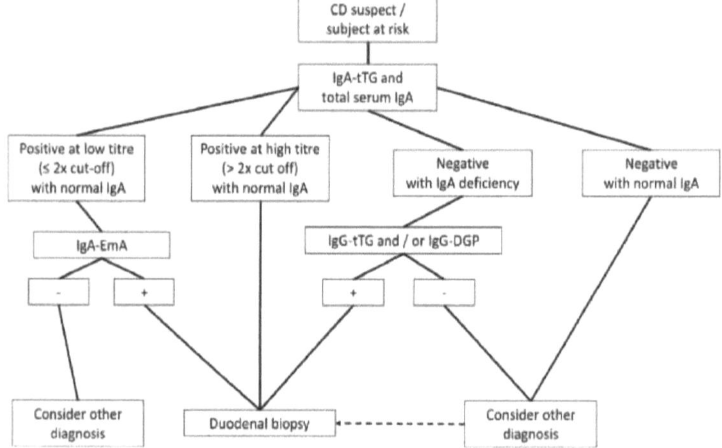

CD: *Celiac disease*; IgA: immunoglobulin A; tTG: tissue transglutaminase; DGP: *Deamidated Gliadin Peptide*; +: Positive; -: Negative

Figure 14: Diagnostic algorithm for coeliac disease in adults [6].

2. CURRENT TREATMENT FOR COELIAC DISEASE

Currently, the only effective treatment available for CD is a strict, lifelong GFD. In the majority of cases, this diet resolves both intestinal and extra-intestinal symptoms, and enables negative results to be obtained when autoantibodies are tested. It also encourages the regrowth of intestinal villi. This diet offers protection against the various complications of CD. Although dietary gluten restriction is a safe and effective therapy, accidental exposure to gluten in the context of a GFD is common. Theoretically, the introduction of a GFD may seem fairly straightforward, but in practice it is very restrictive [6,59].

2.1.Gluten-free diet

2.1.1. Definition of a gluten-free product

The Codex Alimentarius of the World Health Organisation has regulated the content of gluten-free products to guarantee the safety of people following a GFD. In order to be declared gluten-free, a product must have a gluten content of less than 20 mg/kg. However, these levels vary from country to country [60]. According to European Union regulations on gluten-free products, if the amount of gluten is between 21 mg/kg and 100 mg/kg, the product can be labelled as having a very low gluten content [61].

Identifying gluten in gluten-free products is often complex and can be overlooked, particularly when terms such as 'modified wheat starch' are used. It is therefore essential that consumers have some nutritional knowledge to detect these ingredients. To help with this identification task, the UK Coeliac Association has pioneered the creation of the crossed-out wheat ear logo **(Figure 15)**. This logo has been certified and protected by the *Association of European Coeliac Societies* (AOECS) since 1995, guaranteeing the total absence of gluten in industrial products [62].

Figure 15: The crossed wheat ear logo of the *Association of European Coeliac Societies* (AOECS) [63].

Many foods are naturally gluten-free and can therefore be eaten without restriction by people with CD. Fruit, vegetables, meat, fish, eggs, dairy products, oils and nuts are all naturally gluten-free. In addition, alternative cereals that are safe to eat include rice, maize, quinoa and buckwheat. Legumes such as lentils, chickpeas and beans can also be eaten **(Table IV)**. These foods are an important source of essential nutrients such as fibre, vitamins and minerals, offering a healthy and safe alternative for coeliac patients **[64]**.

Table IV: Cereals and pseudocereals authorised and not authorised in the gluten-free diet (according to [65]).

PermitNo	Permit	
Cereals	-Maize -Rice -Sorghum -Oats *	-Wheat (spelt, semolina, durum) -Rye -Barley -Kamut®
Pseudocereals	-Buckwheat -Quinoa -Amaranth	

* Always a subject of debate

2.1.2. History of the gluten-free diet

In 1887, the English physician Samuel Gee was one of the first authors to describe the GFD **[66]**. However, it was the Dutch doctor Willem Karel Dicke who really brought the benefits of this diet to light and who noted an improvement in patients who excluded gluten from their diet. In fact, Dr Dicke observed that the health of coeliac children improved considerably when wheat, rye and barley were removed from their staple diet following their shortage in the Netherlands during the Second World War, only to relapse at the end of the war when wheat flour was reintroduced. Following this, he proposed a cereal-free diet to treat his CD patients **[67]**. In Europe, paediatricians were the first to come into contact with CD patients despite the fact that, at that time, knowledge of CD and the GFD was limited, even among healthcare professionals. Providing advice on GFD to diagnosed children and their parents was a challenge, as there were no gluten-free products on the market and the necessary information for manufacturers was scarce. Gluten-free bread and gluten-free flour were the most sought-after products. Professionals recommended mixing potato and maize flour to make gluten-free bread. Soya flour was used as an alternative for making cakes and desserts. Unfortunately, these types of flour were rare, which made it difficult to produce gluten-free foods. It is important to note that, even before the establishment of specialist organisations, mothers of children with CD took the initiative by establishing contacts between parents and forming informal groups. This growing demand for GSRs eventually led to the creation of private companies producing gluten-free products **[68]**.

2.1.3. Benefits of the gluten-free diet

2.1.3.1. Reduction in symptoms associated with coeliac disease

The inflammation of the small intestine caused by CD gives rise to a variety of unpleasant symptoms. Adopting a GFD offers coeliac patients the chance to reduce these symptoms considerably. Eliminating gluten from the diet reduces abdominal pain, bloating and bowel problems such as diarrhoea and constipation. Clinical studies have confirmed an improvement in symptoms in coeliac patients who follow a rigorous GFD. This dietary change enables patients to regain digestive comfort and improve their quality of life. In 2019, a study demonstrated an increase in height and weight growth with significant catch-up growth in paediatric patients following a strict GFD for two years [69]. Untreated CD is associated with a high prevalence of low bone mineral density, which improves significantly after adherence to the GFD in both adults and children. The GFD also reduces the risk of infertility, spontaneous abortion, premature delivery and low birth weight infants in women with CD. Adherence to a GFD also helps restore the histological architecture of the small intestine and prevents the lymphoproliferative complications of CD [8].

2.1.3.2. Nutritional benefits and dietary diversity

Adherence to a strict GFD can have significant nutritional benefits for people with CD. By avoiding gluten-containing foods, these patients have the opportunity to explore new sources of nutrient-rich foods to ensure a balanced and varied diet. The GFD increases consumption of fruit, vegetables and dairy products. These foods are naturally gluten-free and rich in vitamins, minerals, fibre and antioxidants essential to a healthy diet [70].

2.1.4. Challenges of a gluten-free diet

Increasing adherence to the GFD among CD patients reflects the appeal of the benefits of this diet. However, it is essential that the risks associated with this nutritional approach are considered and not overlooked [71].

2.1.4.1. Unintentional gluten contamination

Joining a GSR represents a radical lifestyle change that can pose many challenges. The threat of cross-contamination is a daily problem for people following a GFD. Several studies based on nutritional questionnaires, serological tests and assessments of immunogenic gluten peptides in stool and urine have reported variable rates of gluten exposure in CD patients, reaching up to 69% in adults, 64% in adolescents and 45% in children, despite their efforts to avoid gluten consumption. Many restaurants offer gluten-free alternatives to meet the growing demand from people following a GFD. However, a recent study in 2019 revealed that up to 32% of foods labelled gluten-free in restaurants tested positive for gluten. These results highlighted the need for additional precautions when selecting and consuming gluten-free foods outside the home [59,72].

2.1.4.2. Toxic effects of the gluten-free diet

There are two main sources of toxic and potentially dangerous substances in GSR. Certain foods frequently consumed as part of the GFD, such as rice and fish, may contain toxic heavy metals. These contaminants, such as lead, cadmium, mercury and arsenic, can come from a variety of sources, including the environment, farming practices and food processing. Regular consumption of these contaminated foods can lead to an accumulation of these heavy metals in the body, which can have harmful consequences for health, including neurological and kidney disorders and even carcinogenic effects [73]. In addition, the incorporation of food additives into gluten-free products has raised scientific concerns about their safety and potential health effects. Among these additives, microbial TG is widely used to improve the quality of gluten-free products. This microbial TG functionally mimics TG2, which is the autoantigen of CD. The modifications induced by this enzyme can increase the immunogenicity of gluten peptides, thereby increasing the risk of triggering immune reactions and acting as an environmental factor favouring the development of CD in genetically predisposed individuals [74].

2.1.4.3. Nutritional deficiencies and constipation

Nutritional deficiencies and intestinal transit problems can result from poorly managed GFDs (Table V).

Table V: Nutritional problems in patients with

coeliac disease

following a gluten-free diet (after [75]).

Nutritional problems in coeliac patients	
Fat	High intake of fat and saturated fatty acids
Carbohydrates	Low in complex carbohydrates but high in simple sugars
Fibres	Low fibre intake
Vitamins	Low intake of vitamins D, E and B group vitamins (B1, B2, B6, B9, B12)
Minerals	Low intake of iron, calcium, magnesium, zinc, iodine, potassium, selenium and manganese

Gluten-free products generally have different nutritional characteristics to those containing gluten. These products generally contain more fat, sugar or salt (depending on the type of product) than products containing gluten. This exposes the patient to several macronutrient and micronutrient deficiencies and to excessive consumption of fats and carbohydrates [76]. Studies of the nutritional profiles of gluten-free versus gluten-containing products have shown that gluten-free foods are low in fibre, protein, folate, iron, potassium and zinc, and high in fat, carbohydrate and sodium. This could explain the increased incidence of metabolic syndrome and cardiovascular morbidity reported in CD patients on this diet. These nutritional deficiencies may be at the root of the development of severe short- and long-term complications **(Figure 16) [71,77]**.

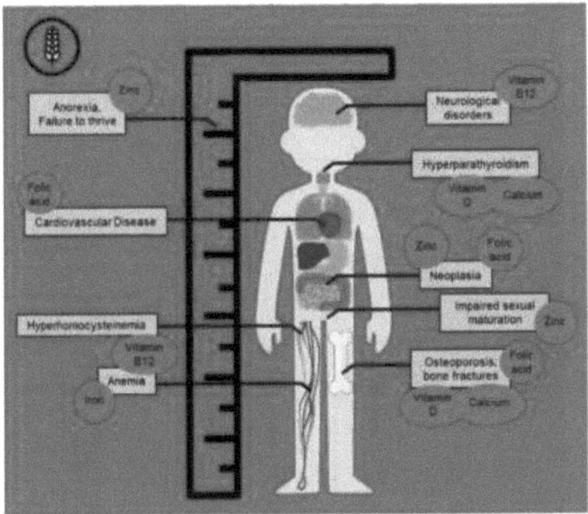

Figure 16: Co-morbidities associated with nutritional deficiencies frequently observed in coeliac patients on a gluten-free diet
[77].

Some studies have shown that gluten-free foods, particularly the substitutes used in the GFD, contain lower levels of fibre than those containing gluten, which often puts people on the GFD at risk of constipation. It is therefore essential that people with CD following a GFD ensure that they include sources of fibre in their diet by consuming foods that are naturally gluten-free and high in fibre, such as fruit, vegetables and pulses **[71,78]**.

2.1.4.4.   Negative impact on quality of life

Strict restrictions on dietary options can lead to a deterioration in the quality of life of coeliac patients, psychological problems and social isolation **(figure17)**.

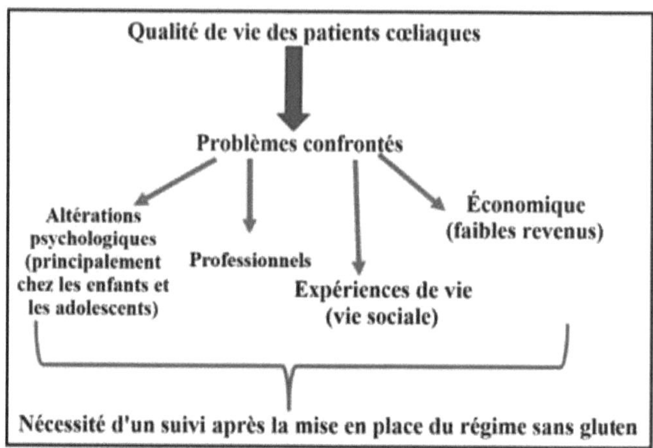

The need for follow-up after the gluten-free diet has been introduced

2.1.4.5.   17: Effect of coeliac disease and gluten-free diet on patients' quality of life [79].

Studies of CD patients on a strict GFD have shown high levels of social isolation and depression. In reality, patients on a GFD have a limited choice of foods and suffer from difficulties in finding gluten-free products. The cost associated with GFD also represents one of the major challenges for people with CD. Indeed, most gluten-free alternatives require additional processing to remove the gluten protein. These high costs can be a considerable financial burden for people following this diet [71].

2.1.5. Resistance to the gluten-free diet

GFR resistance in patients with CD is defined as the absence of improvement or recurrence of clinical and histological signs after 12 months of strict adherence to the GFR. Resistance to GFR can take two forms: primary resistance, which is observed immediately, or secondary resistance, which occurs after an initial positive response to the regimen [8]. In the event of persistent or worsening symptoms and villous atrophy despite adherence to a strict GFD, the clinician should consider

diagnosis of refractory CD **(figure 18) [55, 80]**.

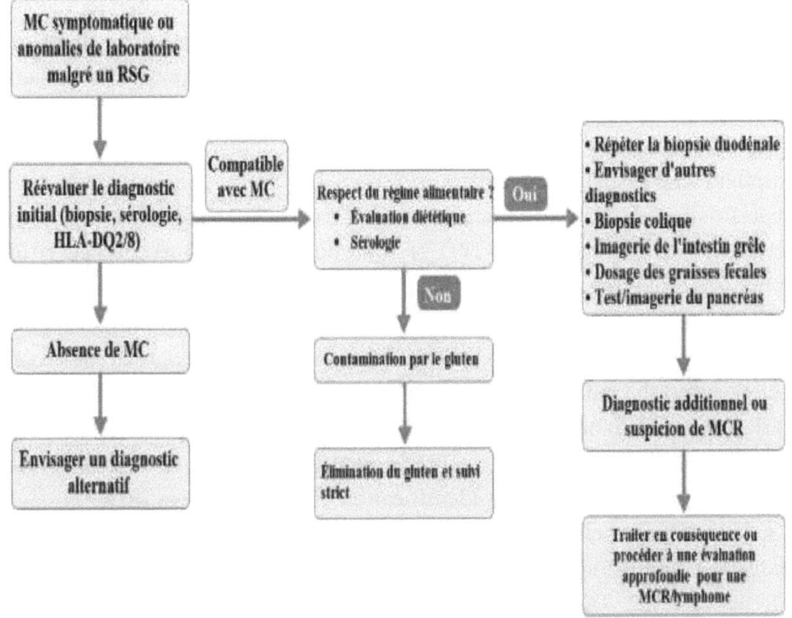

CD: Celiac disease; RSG: Gluten-free diet; HLA: *Human Leukocyte Antigen*; RCM: Refractory celiac disease ;

Figure 18: Diagnostic algorithm for persistent symptoms or histological and serological abnormalities [8].

The management of refractory CD is difficult. Treatment depends largely on the type of disease [8,80]:

• Type I: The main treatment is nutritional support and corticosteroids or immunosuppressants such as azathioprine in the case of cortico-resistance. In the majority of cases, maintenance of a strict GFD plus nutritional support has led to symptomatic and histological improvement.

• Type II: It is recommended that treatment be initiated with prednisolone or budesonide in combination with cladribine. However, immunosuppressive drugs are not recommended as they increase the risk of developing enteropathy-associated T-cell lymphoma (EATL). The use of immunosuppressive chemotherapy followed by haematopoietic stem cell transplantation is rarely used.

2.1.6. Compliance

Regular monitoring of coeliac patients is essential to improve adherence to the GFD. The main objectives of follow-up are to ensure the absence of symptoms and healing of the intestinal mucosa. During the first year after starting the GFD, frequent monitoring is essential to encourage adherence to the diet and to provide psychological support and help patients acclimatise to their new situation. Thereafter, once the disease has stabilised and the patient is managing the GFD without difficulty, annual or biennial follow-ups are recommended. During these consultations, the doctor assesses the integrity of small intestinal absorption, looks for liver disorders and associated autoimmune disorders such as type 1 diabetes and autoimmune thyroid disease, and checks the levels of CD-specific antibodies such as anti-TG2 or AAE and/or anti-PD antibodies. If liver enzyme abnormalities are present, close monitoring at is required. If these abnormalities persist, further evaluation (immunological, radiological and/or histopathological) is recommended [8]. It is essential to emphasise the role of the dietician in the management of CD, so that patients learn not only to follow the GFD, but also to balance it. Dietetic consultation with a dietician specialised in the treatment of CD has been shown to significantly improve adherence to the GFD, mainly through the proper identification of gluten sources [81].

2.2. Education of coeliac patients

Therapeutic education of coeliac patients is a key element in improving adherence to the GFD, thereby relieving gastrointestinal discomfort and improving patients' quality of life **(Figure 19)**. A recent survey [82] highlighted a lack of knowledge among coeliac patients about the disease and the GFD. Hence the need to develop educational programmes and resources to help them manage their diet. Associations supporting people with CD, as well as healthcare professionals and communities, need to collaborate and pool their efforts to develop appropriate educational resources for coeliac patients. Raising awareness helps motivate these patients to adhere to a strict GFD. Educational programmes and resources need to be developed and made available to meet the needs of these patients. Education also helps patients to understand which foods to avoid, to identify hidden sources of gluten and to learn how to cook gluten-free meals. These skills increase their independence and their ability to lead a normal daily life despite dietary constraints. In addition, appropriate education can help reduce the expense of managing CD by avoiding costly dietary errors and improving the patient's overall health, which will reduce the need for healthcare in the long term [83].

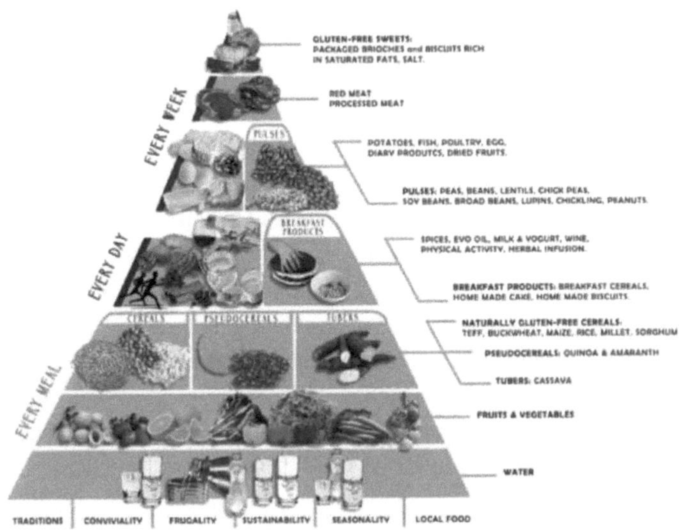

Figure 19: The food pyramid for a gluten-free diet [70].

The integration of *e-learning* can be a means of increasing awareness of the GFD. A study by Connan et al **[84]** highlighted the benefits of interactive online programmes in improving adherence to the GFD and patient knowledge. These online educational programmes include resources such as explanatory videos, interactive quizzes and assessments to measure patient progress. They provide patients with the opportunity to receive accurate, comprehensive and easily accessible information about the RSG at any time. E-learning thus promotes a better understanding of CD and the associated dietary recommendations **(Figure 20) [84]**.

3. NEW THERAPEUTIC APPROACHES TO COELIAC DISEASE

The standard treatment for CD is to eliminate gluten from the diet. This diet is recognised as being highly effective in restoring the integrity of the duodenal mucosa, improving the clinical symptoms of CD and preventing numerous complications. It is often considered by the majority of patients as a constraint, leading to feelings of frustration and having a negative impact on their quality of life. The increasing prevalence of CD, the dissatisfaction of patients with the GFD and the difficulties associated with this regimen have led researchers to explore new therapeutic approaches [85]. The development of new therapies has offered hope that patients can return to a normal diet and enjoy a better quality of life. However, the safety and efficacy of these approaches need to be proven [86].

3.1. Therapies targeting immunogenic epitopes in gluten

Gluten proteins are characterised by a high concentration of proline (15% of the amino acid composition) and glutamine (representing 35% of the amino acid composition). These characteristics confer resistance to intestinal proteases and lead to the production of immunogenic peptides, which can be as long as 30 to 40 amino acids. It is these large peptides that are responsible for the immune response observed in CD patients. Scientists are currently exploring strategies to produce non-immunogenic gluten variants or to neutralise immunogenic gluten peptides [87].

3.1.1. Dietary therapies: Production of non-immunogenic gluten

3.1.1.1. Genetically modified wheat

This strategy involves genetically modifying wheat to make it a non-immunogenic variety, without altering its viscoelastic properties. However, this transformation is complex, as around 100 genes code for gluten, and the inactivation of a single gene would not be enough to achieve the objective. In most cases, inactivation of the genes responsible for gluten immunogenicity has affected its viscoelastic properties [88]. Despite these difficulties, successful transformations have been reported. A transgenic wheat line called E82 has been produced using *RNA interference* (RNAi) technology, which blocks the gliadin genes **(Figure 21)** [88]. A study of 21 CD patients who consumed E82 wheat showed decreased IFN-γ production by peripheral blood mononuclear cells and very low levels of immunogenic gluten peptides in stool samples from these patients, suggesting low exposure to immunogenic epitopes [89].

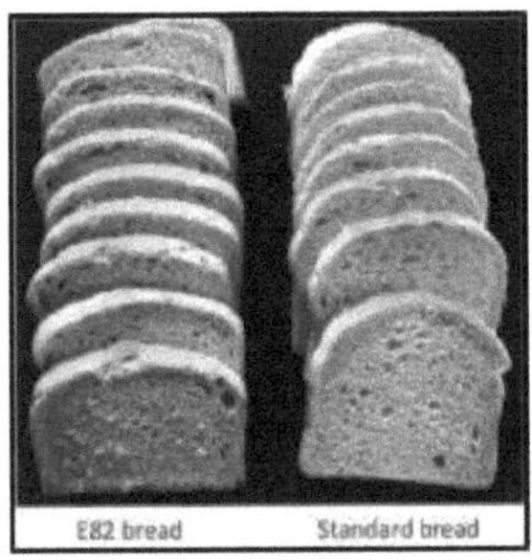

Figure 21: Bread made from E82 flour and standard bread [89].

Prolamins from a wheat variant called C173, obtained by primarily removing toxic epitopes from gliadin fractions, were subjected to in vitro testing on intestinal epithelial cells derived from CD patients. The results showed that there was no worsening of the villi/crypts ratio, but there was an increase in proinflammatory cytokines such as IFNγ and TNF-α, as well as elevated levels of anti-TG2 antibodies in the culture medium [90].

3.1.1.2.   Enzymatic modification of gluten

• **Modification of gluten by proteases**

This approach involves modifying wheat flour by fermentation with bacteria or fungi. The proteolytic enzymes released by these organisms digest the gluten, making it less toxic. However, this transformation alters the texture of the flour. To restore its viscoelastic properties, this flour can be combined with other types of flour such as buckwheat, millet or amaranth [90] . Degradation of the toxic 33-mer peptide, the most immunogenic gliadin peptide responsible for triggering CD, was possible by fermenting sprouted seeds using specific strains of sourdough lactic acid bacteria (such as *Lactobacillus brevis*, *Lactobacillus plantarum* and *Lactobacillus pentosus*). However, these products cannot be considered safe for CD patients, as the daily gluten intake must be between 10 mg/kg and 20 mg/kg. Although this method may have contributed to a significant degradation of the gluten network, the levels achieved were not sufficient to guarantee the safety of food products for people with CD [91]. A 2018 study found that adding wheat flour modified with alanyl aminopeptidase (AnPEP) to a mixture of amaranth flour was an excellent option for obtaining low-gluten bread without additives while preserving satisfactory taste quality. However, further studies are needed to confirm the safety of using this flour in patients with CD [92].

• **Modification of gluten using transglutaminase**

Another enzymatic approach that has been studied to reduce the immunogenicity of gluten is the use of microbial TG extracted from

Streptoverticillium mobaraensis. Although it has the same site of action as human TG, microbial TG lacks deamidation activity and is not calcium-dependent. In vitro studies, animal studies and in vivo studies on intestinal explants from CD patients have suggested a reduction in the immunogenicity of gliadin in wheat flour modified with microbial TG. In a phase 2 clinical trial involving seven CD patients in remission, it was observed that two patients who consumed modified wheat versus four patients who consumed unmodified wheat for 90 days showed an increase in CD-specific antibodies and one versus four showed villous deterioration. Research was carried out to determine whether the peptide end products of gluten transamidated by this enzyme had immunotoxicity similar to that of human TG products. The results showed that microbial TG increased deamidation products by 70% at 40°C and neutral pH. Consequently, the safety of using microbial TG in celiac disease remains uncertain [90].

3.1.1.3. Thermally modified wheat gluten

Researchers have developed an innovative technology using microwaves to detoxify gluten proteins in wheat. The technology involves placing clean, 18-20% hydrated wheat grains in a microwave oven at 1000 watts for 2 minutes prior to grinding, in order to rapidly reach a high temperature of around 110°C to 120°C. The grains are then dried at room temperature (24°C) for 12 to 24 hours and milled to obtain flour. This process has been suggested to reduce gluten immunotoxicity by 99%. The treatment of wheat grains by micro wave will enable the hydrogen bonds between glutamine residues to be broken, thereby promoting conformational and/or structural changes in proteins [93]. According to a study carried out in 2021, microwave detoxification of gluten can be used as a pre-treatment prior to enzymatic hydrolysis. The results of the study showed a modification of the structure of the gluten as well as its immunogenicity. The use of a combination of enzymatic hydrolysis and microwave pre-treatment (200 watts, 100°C, 1 minute) proved effective in reducing gluten content, resulting in an approximately 10-fold decrease in immunogenic epitopes detected by ELISA using the R5 antibody. Future research and clinical trials are needed to better understand the mechanism of inactivation of toxic gluten epitopes by this combined approach [94].

3.1.2. Non-dietary therapies: Blocking exposure to immunogenic gluten

In order to trigger an immune response, gluten must cross the intestinal epithelial barrier and reach the lamina propria. Strategies have been proposed to neutralise gluten after dietary exposure before it is presented to the immune system by APCs [87].

3.1.2.1. Intraluminal digestion of gluten using exogenous endopeptidases

Gluten proteins, rich in proline and glutamine, are known to be resistant to the action of human intestinal proteases. New strategies aim to overcome this problem. They involve the oral administration of exogenous endopeptidases, which have the ability to digest gluten proteins into non-immunogenic peptides before they reach the duodenum. To be able to use them, these enzymes must meet several criteria:

* The ability to break down the various immunogenic sequences of gluten
* Be stable and active in the acidic environment of the stomach and escape degradation by gastric proteases
* The absence of adverse effects in the patient

Several micro-organisms have been identified for their ability to express prolyl-endopeptidases, such as *Aspergillus niger* and *Flavobacterium meningosepticum*. These enzymes have been shown to degrade gluten proteins in vitro and in vivo **(Figure 22)**.

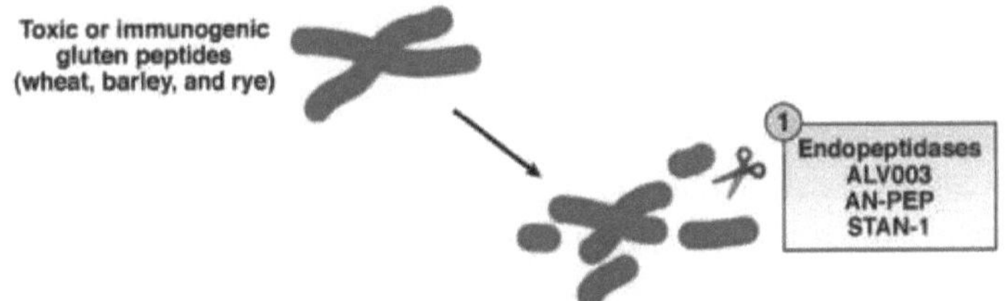

Figure 22: Breakdown of gluten into non-immunogenic peptides by

various endopeptidases [95].

Latiglutenase is currently the most widely studied drug for treating CD **(Table VI)**. It is a mixture of two gluten proteases: ALV001 (a modified recombinant version of glutamine endopeptidase EP-B2) and ALV002 (a modified recombinant version of prolyl-endopeptidase from *Sphingomonas capsulata*) **[87,95]**.

Table VI: The various clinical trials conducted on latiglutenase.

Study	Test phase	Population	Treatment	Duration	Main results (compared with placebo)
Tye-Din, 2010 [96]	1	20 CD patients exposed to a gluten-containing diet (16g/day)	800 mg/day vs placebo	3 days	- Decreased secretion of INF-γ by gluten-specific LTs in peripheral blood
Lahdeaho, 2014 [97]	2a	41 CD patients exposed to a gluten-containing diet (2 g/day)	900 mg/day vs placebo	6 weeks	• Prevention of deterioration of the intestinal mucosa (no decrease in the

					villi/crypts ratio or increase in LELs) • No improvement in symptoms
Murray, 2017 [98];	2b	494 CD patients with moderate or severe symptoms on a GFD $\geq$ 1 year	100 mg, 300 mg, 450 mg, 600 mg, or 900 mg/day vs placebo	12 or 24 weeks	• No difference in villi/crypts ratio or increase in LEL. • No difference in serology
Syage, 2017 [99]	2b	398 seropositive and seronegative CD patients on a GFD $\geq$ 1 year	100 mg, 300 mg, 450 mg, 600 mg, or 900 mg/day vs placebo	12 weeks	- Improvement in symptoms in HIV-positive patients
Murray, 2022 [100]	2b	43 CD patients exposed to a gluten-containing diet (2 g/day)	200 mg/day vs placebo	6 weeks	• Prevention of damage to the intestinal mucosa • Tendency for symptoms to diminish
NCT 04243551 [101]	2b	120 symptomatic CD patients treated with RSG with periodic exposure to gluten	Daily oral administration vs. placebo	6 weeks	In progress Estimated completion December 2023

CD: Coeliac disease; RSG: Gluten-free diet; INF-γ: Interferon gamma; LT: T lymphocyte; LIE: Lymphocytes intraepithelial; NCT: *National Clinical Trial*.

Another study investigating the efficacy of prolyl-endopeptidase (AN-PEP), derived from *Aspergillus niger*, also showed a capacity to degrade gluten in vitro **(Table VII) [87]**. More recently, a study carried out in 2021 showed that TAK-62, a glutenase effective in vitro, was well tolerated and capable of degrading up to 97% of the gluten in gastric aspirates from patients with CD **(Table VII) [102]**.

Table VII: Various clinical trials conducted on AN-PEP and TAK-62.

Agent	Study	Test phase	Population	Treatment	Duration	Main results (vs Placebo)
AN PEP	Tack, 2013 [103]	2	14 CD patients exposed to a gluten-containing diet (7 g/day)	Administration of either ANPEP or placebo	2 weeks	- No difference in villi/crypts ratio or LEL increase - No difference observed in terms of quality of life
	NCT 04788 797 [104]	4	40 CD patients treated with RSG exposed to a gluten-containing diet	2 capsules/ day vs placebo	8 weeks	Completed December 2022 No data published
TAK-062	Pultz, 2021	1	139 CD patients	100-900mg vs placebo	6 weeks	- Well tolerated and breaks down large

| [105] | | following a GFD and healthy subjects after a meal containing 3 to 9 g of gluten | | | quantities of gluten quickly and efficiently |

CD: Celiac disease; RSG: Gluten-free diet; IEL: Intraepithelial lymphocytes; NCT: *National Clinical Trial*.

3.1.2.2. Intraluminal sequestration of gluten immunogenic epitopes

This strategy involves trapping and neutralising gluten proteins in the intestinal lumen, thereby preventing their digestion into immunogenic gluten peptides. Two main therapies have been studied [87,90]:

- AGY is a polyclonal anti-gliadin antibody. In vitro tests showed that gliadin absorption was reduced. In fact, it fell from 42.8% to 0.7% with the addition of AGY. AGY was then tested in a clinical trial to verify its safety **(Table VIII)**.

Table VIII: Various clinical trials conducted on AGY

Study	Test phase	Population	Treatment	Duration	Main results
Sample, 2017 [106]	1	10 CD patients undergoing RSG	1000 mg twice vs placebo	4 weeks	• Reduction in symptoms. • Negativation of serology. • LMER* reduction
NCT 03707730 [107]	2	149 CD patients on a GFD who continue to have recurrent symptoms	1 capsule/day before meals vs placebo	14 weeks	Completed in December 2022 No data published

CD: Celiac disease; RSG: Gluten-free diet; LMER: *lactulose: mannitol excretion ratio*; NCT: *National Clinical Trial*.

LMER*: is a quantitative assay that measures the ability of two non-metabolised sugar molecules, lactulose and mannitol, to cross the intestinal mucosa. Mannitol, an easily absorbed monomer, serves as a marker of transcellular absorption, while lactulose, a poorly absorbed dimer, serves as a marker of mucosal integrity. A high lactulose/mannitol ratio is an indicator of intestinal barrier dysfunction.

- BL-7010 is a non-absorbable, high molecular weight copolymer of hydroxyethylmethacrylate and styrene sulphonate - P(HEMA-co-SS). In vitro studies have demonstrated the polymer's high affinity for gliadin, as well as its ability to heal gluten-induced intestinal lesions in in vivo mouse models. In addition, the use of this copolymer resulted in a reduction in TNF-α secretion in mucosal biopsies taken from CD patients in the presence of partially digested gliadin. A clinical trial was completed in 2014 in coeliac patients, but no data have been published **(Figure 23, Table VIII)**.

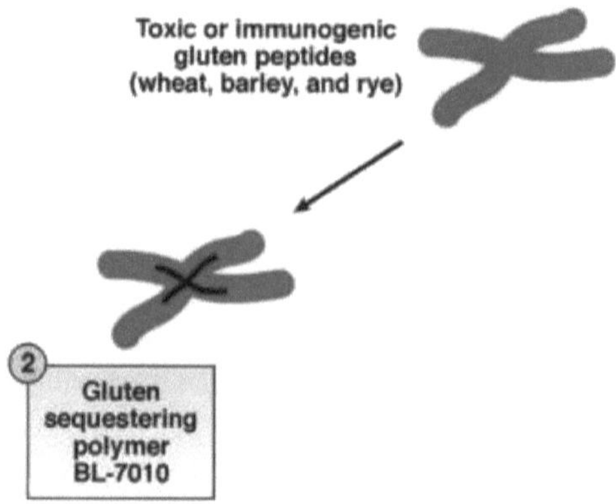

Figure 23: BL7010, binds to intraluminal gliadin, preventing its release and degradation into immunogenic peptides [95].

Table IX: Various clinical trials conducted on BL-7010.

Study	Phase test	Population	Treatment	Duration	Main results
NCT 01990885 [108]	1	40 CD patients undergoing RSG	The study is in two parts: -Part A: Patients will receive a single dose of BL-7010. -Part B: Patients will receive three doses of BL-7010 or placebo.	14 days	Completed in 2014 No data published

CD: Celiac disease; RSG: Gluten-free diet; NCT: *National Clinical Trial*

3.1.2.3. Decreased epithelial permeability

Impaired paracellular permeability is an early event in the development of CD, allowing immunogenic gluten peptides to pass through this pathway. Zonulin, expressed in large quantities in the intestinal mucosa and blood of CD patients, is an enzyme that regulates epithelial permeability. Binding of gliadin to the chemokine receptor CXCR3 results in the release of zonulin, which increases intestinal permeability via the MyD88-dependent pathway. Zonulin shares a structural similarity with the zonula occludens toxin produced by *Vibrio cholerae* **[87,90]**. Strategies targeting tight junctions have been developed to modulate intestinal permeability to gluten. Larazotide acetate is a synthetic octapeptide structurally related to the zonula occludens toxin produced by the bacterium *Vibrio cholera*. This drug improves the function of the intestinal barrier by inhibiting the action of zonulin by blocking its receptor. Several clinical trials have been conducted with larazotide to assess its efficacy in modulating tight junctions and intestinal permeability to gluten **(Figure 24, Table IX)**. However, strategies aimed at reducing intestinal permeability are hampered by pathways

transcellular passages that allow the gluten to pass from the light to the cell wall.
lamina propria [87].

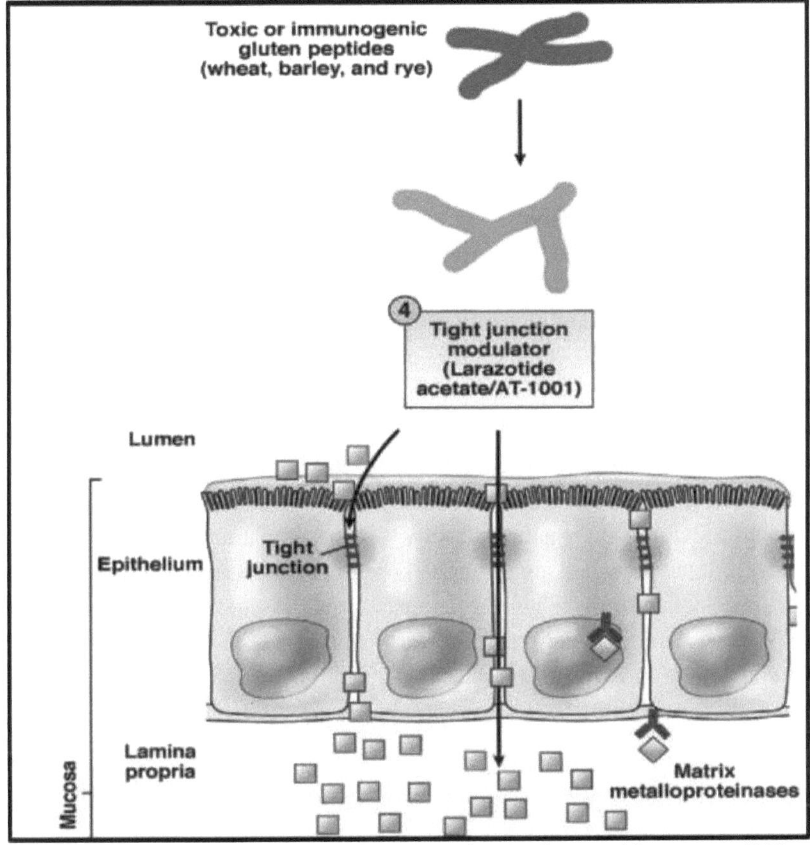

Figure 24: Modulation of the tight junction by larazotide acetate [95].

Table X: Different clinical trials conducted on larazotide acetate

Study	Phase test	Population	Treatment	Duration	Main results
Paterson, 2007 [109]	1	21 CD patients exposed to a gluten-containing diet (2.5 g) for one day	12 mg vs placebo	3 days	• Decreased secretion of INF-γ • Improvement in symptoms • No difference in the LMAR
Leffler, 2012 [110]	2a	86 CD patients exposed to a	0.25 mg, 1 mg, 4 mg,	14 days	• Improvement in symptoms

		gluten-containing diet (2.4 g/day)	or 8 mg/day vs placebo		• No difference in the LMAR
Kelly, 2013 **[111]**	2b	177 CD patients exposed to a gluten-containing diet (2.7 g/day)	1 mg, 4 mg, or 8 mg/day vs placebo	6 weeks	• Improvement in symptoms • Negativation of serology • No difference in the LMAR

CD: celiac disease; LMAR: *lactulose:mannitol excretion ratio*; INF-γ: interferon gamma

3.1.2.4. Action of probiotics

Intestinal dysbiosis has been reported in most patients with CD. As a result, probiotics have been proposed as a treatment strategy for CD. Probiotics are live non-pathogenic micro-organisms administered orally in adequate quantities to restore the intestinal microbiota, promote digestion and inhibit colonisation of the gut by pathogenic bacteria responsible for the development of several diseases [112]. A study carried out in 2017 [113] showed that probiotics can increase the concentration of faecal bifidobacteria in coeliac patients without reaching the concentration observed in healthy subjects. Another study [114] also confirmed the enzymatic capacity of certain strains of lactobacilli to hydrolyse gluten peptides, suggesting the use of probiotics as an adjunct to GFD in coeliac patients. A phase 2 clinical trial evaluated the use of the *Bifidobacterium infantis* strain in the treatment of CD **(Figure 25, Table X)**. Probiotics have promising therapeutic potential in the treatment of CD, particularly when combined with an appropriate diet [95].

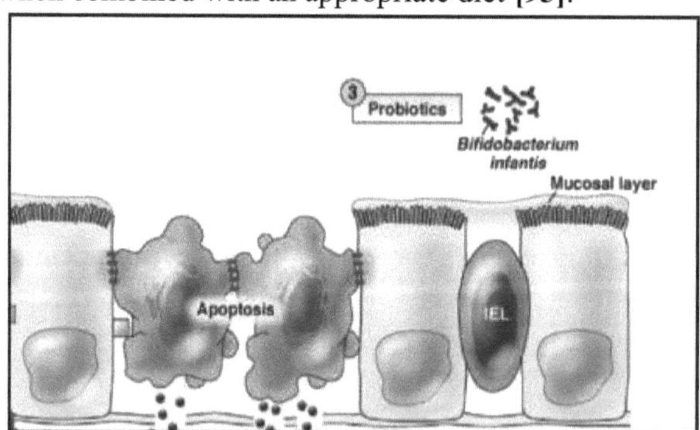

IEL : Intraepithelial lymphocyte

Figure 25: Protection of epithelial cells from gliadin damage by probiotics [95].

Table XI: Clinical trial conducted on probiotics.

Agent	Mechanism action	Clinical trial	Summary of trial results clinic

Bifidobacterium infantis	Protects epithelial cells against damage caused by gliadin	NCT01257620 **[115]**	• Significant improvement in CD symptoms. • The concentrations of anti-TG2 IgA and anti-PDG IgA antibodies at the end of the study, compared with the initial values, were lower in the group treated with *Bifidobacterium infantis* than in the control group. • No change in abnormal intestinal permeability.

CD: Celiac disease; IgA: Immunoglobulin A; TG: Transglutaminase; PDG: Gliadin deamidated peptide; NCT: *National Clinical Trial.*

3.2. Therapies targeting transglutaminase 2 inhibition

TG2 inhibition is one of the promising approaches for the treatment of CD. Recent studies have shown that blocking this enzyme can inhibit gluten-induced immune activation in vitro and in vivo in intestinal biopsies from patients with CD **(Figure 26)**. ZED1227 is an oral selective inhibitor of TG2 **[87]**. Phase 1 clinical trials demonstrated that it was safe and well tolerated in 100 healthy male and female volunteers treated with ZED1227 up to 500 mg **[116]**. Recently, a phase 2 trial **trial [117]** tested increasing doses of ZED1227 (10 mg, 50 mg or 100 mg).

for 6 weeks and compared it with a placebo in 160 coeliac patients on a diet containing 3g of gluten per day. The results showed that use of the 100 mg dose of ZED1227 attenuated villous atrophy and improved symptoms and quality of life in CD patients. Adverse events in all groups included headache, nausea, diarrhoea, vomiting, abdominal pain and rash.

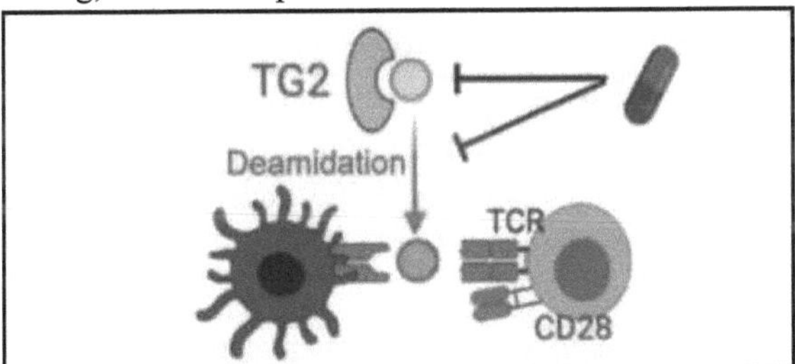

TG: transglutaminase; TCR: *T Cell Receptor*; CD: *cluster of differenciation*

Figure 26: Blockage of deamidation of gluten peptides by the transglutaminase 2 inhibitor [118].

3.3. Therapies targeting immune modulation
3.3.1. Blocking of HLA-DQ2/DQ8 molecules

Approaches aimed at blocking the HLA-DQ2/DQ8 molecules are currently being developed, but remain at a preclinical stage. The aim of these HLA molecule blockers is to prevent the interaction between APCs and CD4+ T *cell* receptors (TCRs), which play a central role in triggering the immunotoxic cascade in CD. One strategy is to use competitive inhibitors in the form of gluten peptide analogues with a higher binding affinity to HLA molecules than gluten. Studies have shown that these inhibitors were able to slightly attenuate LT activation in vitro **(Figure 27)**. However, the use of such therapy remains difficult, particularly because of the rapid degradation of the peptide ligand and possible interference with other vital functions under the immune surveillance of the HLA system **[87,95]**.

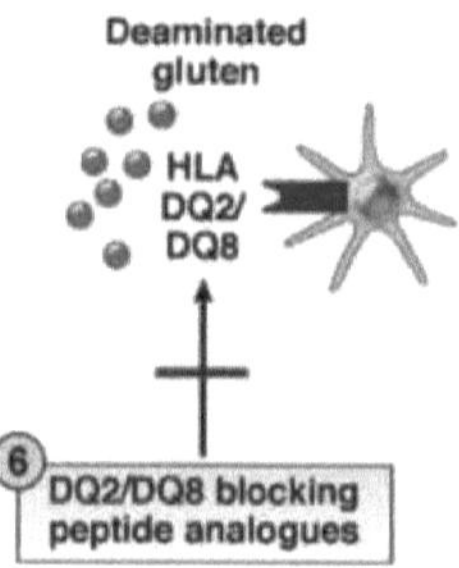

HLA: Human leukocyte antigen
Figure 27: Blockade of HLA DQ2/DQ8 molecules by peptide analogues preventing T cell activation [95].

3.3.2. Inhibition of lymphocyte infiltration

This therapeutic approach involves targeting adhesion molecules on intestinal endothelial cells (*"Mucosal vascular addressin cell adhesion molecule 1"* (MAdCAM 1), as well as their homologous integrin receptors on lymphocytes (integrin receptor α4β7), and tissue-specific chemokine receptors on lymphocytes (chemokine receptor-9, CCR9) **[87]**.

Several therapeutic molecules targeting α4β7 and CCR9 receptors have been studied in order to block lymphocyte migration towards the intestine **(Table XI)**.

PTG-100 is an orally administered α4β7 peptide antagonist. Its use showed a dose-dependent improvement in intestinal lesions in patients with ulcerative colitis in a phase 2a clinical trial **[119]**. Vedolizumab, an anti-α4β7 monoclonal antibody, was evaluated in a phase 2 clinical trial in patients with CD, but showed a lack of efficacy. Finally, vercirnon, an oral selective CCR9 antagonist, initially showed promising results in the treatment of Crohn's disease, but in a phase 3 clinical trial this treatment failed to demonstrate efficacy. A phase 2 study of vercirnon in coeliac patients was completed in 2008, but the results have not been published [87].

Table XII: Various clinical trials conducted on PTG-100, vedolizumab and vercirnon.

Agent	Study	Phase test	Population	Treatment	Duration	Results main
PTG-100 (anti-α4β7)	NCT 045242 21 [120]	1b	30 CD patients exposed to a gluten-containing diet	600 mg capsules twice a day vs. placebo	42 days	Completed in April 2022 ; No data published
Vedolizumab (anti-α4β7)	NCT 029293 16 [121]	2	CD patients exposed to a gluten-containing diet	300 mg intravenously at weeks 0, 2 and 6	6 weeks	Suspended in 2018 due to a lack of participants
Vercinon CCX282-B (anti-CCR9)	NCT 005406 57 [122]	2	90 CD patients exposed to a gluten-containing diet	250 mg twice daily vs placebo	13 weeks	Completed in 2008 ; No data published

CD: Celiac disease; NCT: *National Clinical Trial*

3.3.3. Inhibition of interleukin 15

IL-15 plays an important role in the pathogenesis of CD. It is produced by both APCs and epithelial cells. Overexpression of IL-15 stimulates the production and proliferation of IELs, thereby promoting villous atrophy.

The IL-15 receptor is made up of three different chains:

- An α chain specific for IL-15 (IL15Rα)
- A β-chain (IL-15Rβ) shared with the IL-2 receptor
- A common cytokine receptor γ chain shared with IL-2, IL-4, IL-7, IL-9 and IL-21 receptors

When IL-15 binds to its receptor, the *"Janus kinase signal transducer and activator of transcription pathway"* (JAK/STAT) signalling pathway is activated. Blocking the action of IL-15 with monoclonal antibodies has been shown to prevent tissue destruction **(Figure 28)** [33,123].

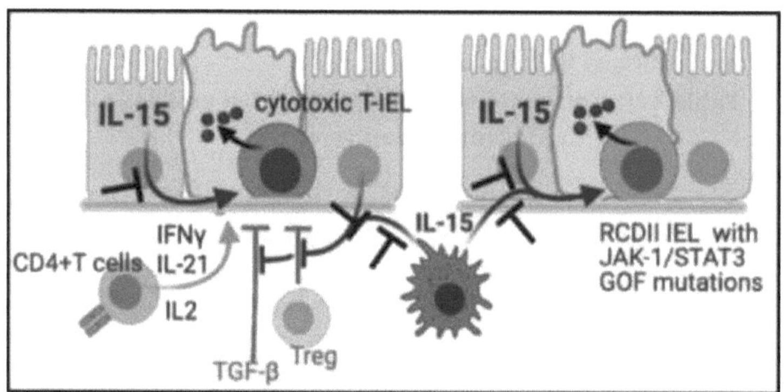

IL: Interleukin; CD: *Cluster of Differentiation*; IFN-γ: Interferon gamma; TGF-β: "RCD: *Refractory celiac disease*; Treg: Regulatory T lymphocytes; IEL: *Intraepithelial lymphocytes*; JAK1: Janus kinase 1; STAT3: *Signal transducer and activator of transcription 3*; GOF mutations: *Gain of Function Mutation*

Figure 28: Prevention of tissue destruction by the antibody monoclonal anti-interleukin 15 [118].

PRN-015, formerly known as AMG714, is the first anti-IL-15 mAb to be evaluated for the treatment of CD. It is a fully human IgG1 monoclonal antibody that binds to IL-15. In clinical trials, treatment with PRN-015 was associated with a reduction in LELs and an improvement in symptoms, but did not alter serological or histological abnormalities in patients with CD. Even in patients with refractory type II CD, it showed no histological benefit. In addition, treatment with PRN-015 has been associated with serious adverse events such as tuberculosis and cerebellar syndrome [124,125].

In an attempt to find effective strategies to treat refractory type II CD, a humanised monoclonal antibody targeting IL-15Rβ which is Hu-Myk- β1 has been explored. However, the results of the phase 1 study conducted to evaluate the efficacy of this antibody have not yet been published [87].

In parallel, preclinical studies in transgenic mice have shown that tofacitinib, an oral JAK inhibitor, has the capacity to improve intestinal lesions in these IL-15 overexpressing mice [126]. In addition, clinical cases have reported significant improvement in histology in patients on a gluten-containing diet, as well as in patients with refractory type II CD. These results led to the initiation of a phase 2 clinical trial currently underway to evaluate the efficacy of tofacitinib in the treatment of refractory type II CD **(Table XII) [127,128]**.

Table XIII: Different clinical trials conducted with PRN-015, Hu-Myk-β1 and tofacitinib.

Agent	Study	Test	Population	Treatment	Duration	Main results

		phase				
PRN-015 or AMG714 (anti-IL-15)	Lähdeaho, 2019 **[129]**	2a	64 CD patients exposed to a gluten-containing diet (2 to 4 g/day)	150 mg, 300 mg/day vs placebo	12 weeks	• Improvement in symptoms (diarrhoea) • Reduction in LELs to 300 mg • No difference in serology or villi/crypts ratio
	Cellier, 2019 **[130]**	2a	MCR Type II	8 mg/kg twice weekly vs placebo	12 weeks	- Improvement in symptoms (diarrhoea) - No difference in the number of LELs, the number of aberrant LELs, or the villi/crypt ratio - Adverse events: 26% vs. 11%.
	NCT 04424927 **[131]**	2b	220 patients with CD resistant to RSG	3 groups receiving different doses (low, medium and high) of sterile solution for subcutaneous administration vs. placebo	28 weeks	In progress, scheduled for completion in December 2023
Hu-Mik-β1 (anti-IL15Rβ1)	NCT 01893775 **[132]**	1	5 patients with RCM	One dose every 3 weeks administered on day 1, week 3 and week 6	9 weeks	Completed December 2019 No data published
Tofacitinib (pan-JAK inhibitor)	Eudra CT: 201800167810 **[133]**	2	Type II RCM patients on a strict GFD	5 to 10 mg	12 weeks	In progress

CD: Celiac disease; GFD: Gluten-free diet; ILL: Intraepithelial lymphocytes; RCM: Refractory celiac disease

3.3.4. Glucocorticoids

Glucocorticoids, including budesonide, are used in the treatment of patients with refractory CD who do not respond to conventional therapies. However, a recent study conducted in 2021 in 27 patients with newly diagnosed CD showed no significant benefit of budesonide as adjuvant therapy to a GFR for healing of the intestinal mucosa. Indeed, remission occurred around the eighth week in about a quarter of patients and was associated with less severe histological lesions at the time of diagnosis **[87,134]**.

3.4. Therapy inducing immune tolerance

CD is marked by a loss of immune tolerance to gluten. Several strategies have been studied to restore tolerance in coeliac patients **[87]**.

3.4.1. Nanoparticles

TAK-101, previously known as TIMP-GLIA, consists of gliadin encapsulated in negatively charged nanoparticles. Following intravenous administration, TAK-101 is taken up by APCs in the liver and spleen, altering their transcription towards anti-inflammatory activity with :

- Inhibition of the co-stimulatory molecules CD80 and CD86.
- Stimulation of the immune checkpoint inhibitor *"Programmed cell Death 1"* (PD-L1).
- Stimulation of the production of the regulatory cytokines IL-10 and TGF-β.

In addition, TAK-101 inhibits the expression of intestinal migration (α4β7) and intestinal retention (αEβ7) integrins in circulating LTs **(Figure 29)**. Recently, a phase 2 study evaluating TAK-101 in 33 CD patients with HLA-DQ2 or 8 and exposed to a gluten-containing diet was conducted. The results showed that TAK-101 was well tolerated and prevented gluten-induced immune activation, thereby inducing specific immune tolerance to gluten. Administration of TAK-101 on days one and eight reduced the growth of an INF-γ-producing cell population by 88% and also inhibited villous flattening compared with placebo. A phase 2 trial is currently underway to determine the optimal doses of TAK-101 in 168 CD patients on a gluten-containing diet. The results of this trial will be available in January 2024 **[87,135]**.

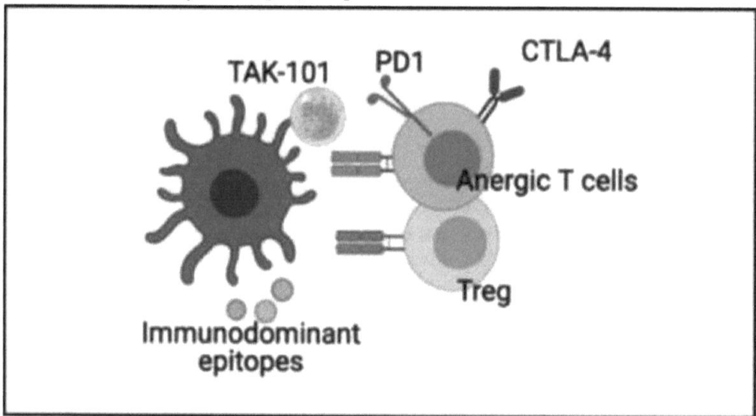

PD1: *Programmed cell death 1*; CTLA-4: *Cytotoxic T lymphocyte antigen 4*; Treg: Regulatory T lymphocytes

Figure 29: Induction of immunotolerance by TAK-101 nanoparticles [118].

3.4.2. Erythrocyte-binding antigens

This approach is currently being developed. It involves combining erythrocytes with fragments of gluten. Red blood cells undergo early apoptosis, leading to their death. These dying erythrocytes, in association with gluten, are then recognised by immune cells, inducing specific tolerance to gluten. KAN-101 is currently the subject of a phase 2 study evaluating its safety **(Table XIII) [87]**.

Table XIV: Clinical trial conducted on KAN-101.

Study	Phase test	Population	Treatment	Duration	Main results
NCT 04248 855 [136]	1	41 CD patients undergoing RSG	The study is in two parts: Part A: Patients will receive a single dose of KAN-101. Part B: Patients will receive three doses of KAN-101 or placebo.	28 days	Completed in October 2021 No data published

CD: Celiac disease; NCT: *National Clinical Trial*

3.4.3. Vaccination

Gluten vaccination is a therapeutic option being considered by researchers to desensitise CD patients to gliadin peptides. Nexvax-2 is a therapeutic vaccine composed of three non-adjuvanted peptides (NPL001, NPL002 and NPL003) containing immunodominant epitopes, aimed at reducing the reactivity of gluten-specific CD4+ LTs. Phase 1 studies showed that Nexvax-2 was well tolerated after intradermal administration, although it caused gastrointestinal symptoms similar to those of gluten exposure, such as diarrhoea and nausea. However, a subsequent phase 1 clinical trial with escalating doses ranging from 60 µg to 150 µg twice weekly for 8 weeks failed to prevent intestinal mucosal deterioration in 108 gluten-exposed CD patients. More recently, a phase 2 study conducted in 2019 with a similar design was stopped prematurely due to vaccine ineffectiveness **[87,95]**.

3.4.4. Treatment with helminths

Inoculation with *Necator americanus*, a type of hookworm, has been studied as a strategy for the treatment of CD. Phase 1 studies showed that inoculation of *Necator americanus* into CD patients exposed to increasing amounts of gluten induced a decrease in INF-γ and IL-17 levels in response to gluten exposure. In addition, this inoculation attenuated the histological and serological abnormalities induced by gluten. However, a phase 2 clinical trial conducted in 2020 showed that *Necator americanus* infestation did not protect patients from gluten-induced mucosal damage and did not restore tolerance to moderate gluten consumption **[87,134]**.

CD is a systemic autoimmune disease affecting the digestive system and affects around 1% of the world's population. It is triggered by the ingestion of gluten, in genetically predisposed individuals. The clinical manifestations of CD vary considerably from patient to patient, including both digestive and extra-digestive symptoms. Currently, the only proven effective treatment for CD is a lifelong GFD, which requires great vigilance and discipline to avoid gluten contamination. GFD is often difficult for patients to follow, as it can lead to nutritional deficiencies and severely restrict their food choices. In addition, some patients may be unable to follow it for medical, psychological or socio-economic reasons. In recent years, the increasing incidence of CD has encouraged the search for new therapeutic strategies to improve the quality of life of patients suffering from CD. The development of new drugs is a complex process that must meet a number of requirements. New treatments must meet a number of criteria, including the absence of serious side effects, simple administration (ideally oral) and reasonable cost. Pharmacological treatments may be particularly useful for CD patients who do not respond to GFR, or as adjuvant treatment in combination with GFR. Two drugs are currently the subject of the most advanced clinical research: larazotide and latiglutenase. Larazotide acts by stabilising enterocyte tight junctions to reduce intestinal permeability. Although clinical trials have not been able to show a reduction in intestinal permeability due to the high variability of the trials, phase 2 studies have shown a reduction in symptoms and serology positivity, suggesting an effective reduction in the amount of gluten to which the immune system is exposed. However, in

2022, a phase 3 trial was suspended after an interim analysis showed a non-significant effect. Latiglutenase is a mixture of glutenases that has shown, in phase 2 studies, the ability to prevent deterioration of the intestinal mucosa and the development of symptoms resulting from exposure to gluten in patients with CD. It is therefore considered to be a promising drug for use as an adjuvant therapy in the treatment of this disease. Patients with refractory CD, or those who do not respond to a GFD, face a therapeutic challenge. Blocking IL-15 with monoclonal antibodies has shown mixed results with potential side effects, while tofacitinib appears more promising by acting on the IL-15 signalling pathway. Strategies for inducing immune tolerance to gluten, such as therapeutic vaccines and hookworm infestation, have so far shown disappointing results.

Thus, the new therapeutic approaches represent a glimmer of hope for patients with CD, and it is essential to continue research in this area. Further studies involving larger populations are needed.

REFERENCES

1. Molder A, Balaban DV, Jinga M, Molder CC. Current evidence on computer-aided diagnosis of celiac disease: Systematic review. Front Pharmacol. 2020;11:341:1-11.

2. Lindfors K, Ciacci C, Kurppa K, Lundin KE, Makharia GK, Mearin ML, et al. Coeliac disease. Nat Rev Dis Primer. 2019;5(1):3 :1-18.

3. Sahin Y. Celiac disease in children: A review of the literature. World J Clin Pediatr. 2021;10(4):**53-71**.

4. Tye-Din JA, Galipeau HJ, Agardh D. Celiac disease: A review of current concepts in pathogenesis, prevention, and novel therapies. Front Pediatr. 2018;6:1-19.

5. Calado J, Verdelho Machado M. Celiac disease revisited. J Gastroenterol. 2022;29(2):**111-24**.

6. Caio G, Volta U, Sapone A, Leffler DA, De Giorgio R, Catassi C, et al. Celiac disease: a comprehensive current review. BMC Med. 2019;17(1):1- 20.

7. Cataldo F, Montalto G. Celiac disease in the developing countries: A new and challenging public health problem.   World J Gastroenterol. 2007;13(15):**2153-9**.

8. Al-Toma A, Volta U, Auricchio R, Castillejo G, Sanders DS, Cellier C, et al. al. European society for the study of coeliac disease (ESsCD) guideline for coeliac disease and other gluten-related disorders. United Eur Gastroenterol J. 2019;7(5):**583-613**.

9. Daly M, Bromilow SN, Nitride C, Shewry PR, Gethings LA, Mills EN. Mapping coeliac toxic motifs in the prolamin seed storage proteins of barley, rye, and oats using a curated sequence database. Front Nutr. 2020;7:1-17.

10. Ahmad I, Swaroop A, Bagchi D. An overview of gluten-free foods and related disorders. In: Bagchi D, editor. Nutraceutical and functional food regulations in the United States and around the world (Third edition). Cambridge: Academic Press; 2019. p. **75-85**.

11. Cárdenas-Torres FI, Cabrera-Chávez F, Figueroa-Salcido OG, Ontiveros N. Non-celiac gluten sensitivity: An update. Medicina. 2021;57(6):1-20.

12. El-Metwally A, Toivola P, AlAhmary K, Bahkali S, AlKhathaami A, AlSaqabi MK, et al. The epidemiology of celiac disease in the general population and high-risk groups in arab countries: A systematic review. Bio Med Res Int. 2020;2020:1-13.

13. Caio G, Volta U, Sapone A, Leffler DA, De Giorgio R, Catassi C, et al. Celiac disease: a comprehensive current review. BMC Med. 2019;17(1):1- 20.

14. Makharia GK, Catassi C. Celiac disease in Asia. Gastroenterol Clin North Am. 2019;48(1):101-13.

15. Sahin Y, Sevinc E, Bayrak NA, Varol FI, Akbulut UE, Bükülmez A. Knowledge regarding celiac disease among healthcare professionals, patients and their caregivers in Turkey. World J Gastrointest Pathophysiol. 2022;13(6):**178-85**.

16. Rubio-Tapia A, Ludvigsson JF, Brantner TL, Murray JA, Everhart JE. The prevalence of celiac disease in the United States. Am J Gastroenterol. 2012;107(10):1538-44.

17. Ben Hariz M, Kallel-Sellami M, Kallel L, Lahmer A, Halioui S, Bouraoui S, et al. Prevalence of celiac disease in Tunisia: mass-screening study in schoolchildren. Eur J Gastroenterol Hepatol. 2007;19(8):**687-94**.

18. King JA, Jeong J, Underwood FE, Quan J, Panaccione N, Windsor JW, et al. Incidence of celiac disease is increasing over time: a systematic review and meta-analysis. Am J Gastroenterol. 2020;115(4):**507-25**.

19. Sahin Y. Celiac disease in children: A review of the literature. World J Clin Pediatr. 2021;10(4):**53-71**.

20. Shewry P. What is gluten-why is it special? Front Nutr. 2019;6:1-10.

21. Pecora F, Persico F, Gismondi P, Fornaroli F, Iuliano S, de'Angelis GL, et al. Gut microbiota in celiac disease: is there any role for probiotics? Front Immunol. 2020;11:1-8.

22. Olshan KL, Leonard MM, Serena G, Zomorrodi AR, Fasano A. Gut microbiota in celiac disease: microbes, metabolites, pathways and therapeutics. Expert Rev Clin Immunol. 2020;16(11):**1075-92**.

23. Caminero A, Galipeau HJ, McCarville JL, Johnston CW, Bernier SP, Russell AK, et al. Duodenal bacteria from patients with celiac disease and healthy subjects distinctly affect gluten breakdown and immunogenicity. Gastroenterology. 2016;151(4):670-83.

24. Szajewska H, Shamir R, Mearin L, Ribes-Koninckx C, Catassi C, Domellöf M, et al. Gluten introduction and the risk of coeliac disease: a position paper by the European society for pediatric gastroenterology, hepatology, and nutrition. J Pediatr Gastroenterol Nutr. 2016;62(3):**507-13**.

25. Martín-Masot R, Diaz-Castro J, Moreno-Fernandez J, Navas-López VM, Nestares T. The role of early programming and early nutrition on the development and progression of celiac disease: A review. nutrients. 2020;12(11):1-18.

26. Caminero A, Verdu EF. Celiac disease: should we care about microbes? Am J Physiol. 2019;317(2):**161-70**.

27. Kahrs CR, Chuda K, Tapia G, Stene LC, Marild K, Rasmussen T, et al. Enterovirus as trigger of coeliac disease: nested case-control study within prospective birth cohort. BMJ. 2019;364:1-8.

28. Sánchez D, Hoffmanová I, Szczepanková A, Hábová V, Tlaskalová-Hogenová H. Contribution of infectious agents to the development of celiac disease. Microorganisms. 2021;9(3):1-21.

29. D'Avino P, Serena G, Kenyon V, Fasano A. An updated overview on celiac disease: from immuno-pathogenesis and immuno-genetics to therapeutic implications. Expert Rev Clin Immunol. 2021;17(3):**269-84**.

30. Brown NK, Guandalini S, Semrad C, Kupfer SS. A clinician's guide to celiac disease HLA genetics. Am J Gastroenterol. 2019;114(10):1587-92.

31. Espino L, Núñez C. The HLA complex and coeliac disease. Int Rev Cell Mol Biol. 2021;358:**47-83**.

32. Wei G, Helmerhorst EJ, Darwish G, Blumenkranz G, Schuppan D. Gluten degrading enzymes for treatment of celiac disease. Nutrients. 2020;12(7):1- 15.

33. Levescot A, Malamut G, Cerf-Bensussan N. Immunopathogenesis and environmental triggers in coeliac disease. Gut. 2022;71(11):**2337-49**.

34. Clément BJ, Lebreton C, Malamut G, Cerf-Bensussan N. Intestinal permeability and celiac disease. Med Mal Metab. 2015;9(1):**19-26**.

35. Tajik N, Frech M, Schulz O, Schälter F, Lucas S, Azizov V, et al. Targeting zonulin and intestinal epithelial barrier function to prevent onset of arthritis. Nat Commun. 2020;11:1-14.

36. Vanuytsel T, Tack J, Farre R. The role of intestinal permeability in gastrointestinal disorders and current methods of evaluation. Front Nutr. 2021;8:1-17.

37. Paolella G, Sposito S, Romanelli AM, Caputo I. Type 2 transglutaminase in coeliac disease: a key player in pathogenesis, diagnosis and therapy. Int J Mol Sci. 2022;23(14):1-25.

38. Yu X, Vargas J, Green PH, Bhagat G. Innate lymphoid cells and celiac disease: current perspective. Cell Mol Gastroenterol Hepatol. 2021;11(3):**803-14**.

39. Voisine J, Abadie V. Interplay between gluten, HLA, innate and adaptive immunity orchestrates the development of coeliac disease. Front Immunol. 2021;12:1-13.

40. Sharma N, Bhatia S, Chunduri V, Kaur S, Sharma S, Kapoor P, et al. Pathogenesis of celiac disease and other gluten related disorders in wheat and strategies for mitigating them. Front Nutr. 2020;7:1-26.

41. Ramírez-Sánchez AD, Tan IL, Gonera-de Jong BC, Visschedijk MC, Jonkers I, Withoff S. Molecular biomarkers for celiac disease: past, present and future. Int J Mol Sci. 2020;21(22):1-25.

42. Dunne MR, Byrne G, Chirdo FG, Feighery C. Coeliac disease pathogenesis: the uncertainties of a well-known immune mediated disorder. Front Immunol.

2020;11:1-14.

43. Ben Houmich T, Admou B. Celiac disease: Understandings in diagnostic, nutritional, and medicinal aspects. Int J Immunopathol Pharmacol. 2021;35:1-22.

44. Ludvigsson JF, Leffler DA, Bai J, Biagi F, Fasano A, Green PH, et al. The Oslo definitions for coeliac disease and related terms. Gut. 2013;62(1):43- 52.

45. Husby S, Koletzko S, Korponay-Szabó I, Kurppa K, Mearin ML, Ribes-Koninckx C, et al. European society paediatric gastroenterology, hepatology and nutrition guidelines for diagnosing coeliac disease 2020. J Pediatr Gastroenterol Nutr. 2020;70(1):**141-56**.

46. Raiteri A, Granito A, Giamperoli A, Catenaro T, Negrini G, Tovoli F. Current guidelines for the management of celiac disease: A systematic review with comparative analysis. World J Gastroenterol. 2022;28(1):154- 75.

47. Leonard MM, Lebwohl B, Rubio-Tapia A, Biagi F. AGA clinical practice update on the evaluation and management of seronegative enteropathies: expert review. Gastroenterology. 2021;160(1):437-44.

48. Therrien A, Kelly CP, Silvester JA. Celiac disease: extraintestinal manifestations and associated conditions. J Clin Gastroenterol. 2020;54(1):**8-21**.

49. Tarar ZI, Zafar MU, Farooq U, Basar O, Tahan V, Daglilar E. The progression of celiac disease, diagnostic modalities, and treatment options. J Investig Med High Impact Case Rep. 2021;9:1-8.

50. Pantic N, Pantic I, Jevtic D, Mogulla V, Oluic S, Durdevic M, et al. Celiac disease and thrombotic events: systematic review of published Cases. Nutrients. 2022;14(10):1-13.

51. Durazzo M, Ferro A, Brascugli I, Mattivi S, Fagoonee S, Pellicano R. Extra-intestinal manifestations of celiac disease: what should we know in 2022? J Clin Med. 2022;11(1):1-15.

52. Roca M, Donat E, Marco-Maestud N, Masip E, Hervás-Marín D, Ramos D, et al. Efficacy study of anti-endomysium antibodies for celiac disease diagnosis: a retrospective study in a spanish pediatric population. J Clin Med. 2019;8(12):1-12.

53. Caetano dos Santos FL, Michalek IM, Laurila K, Kaukinen K, Hyttinen J, Lindfors K. Automatic classification of IgA endomysial antibody test for celiac disease: a new method deploying machine learning. Sci Rep. 2019;9:1-7.

54. Saadah OI, Alamri AM, Al-Mughales JA. Deamidated gliadin peptide and tissue transglutaminase antibodies in children with coeliac disease: A correlation study. Arab J Gastroenterol. 2020;21(3):**174-8**.

55. Bai JC, Ciacci C. World gastroenterology organisation global guidelines. J Clin Gastroenterol. 2017;51(9):**755-68**.

56. Wang X, Qian H, Ciaccio EJ, Lewis SK, Bhagat G, Green PH, et al. Celiac disease diagnosis from videocapsule endoscopy images with residual learning and deep feature extraction. Comput Methods Programs Biomed. 2020;187:1-10.

57. Villanacci V, Vanoli A, Leoncini G, Arpa G, Salviato T, Bonetti LR, et al. Celiac disease: histology-differential diagnosis-complications. A practical approach. Pathologica. 2020;112(3):186-96.

58. Lengliné H, Fabre A. Diagnosis of celiac disease in children. Perfect Pédiatr. 2022;5(2):**2-6**.

59. Segura V, Ruiz-Carnicer Á, Sousa C, Moreno M de L. New insights into non-dietary treatment in celiac disease: emerging therapeutic options. Nutrients. 2021;13(7):1-18.

60. Rodríguez JM, Estévez V, Bascuñán K, Ayala J, Araya M. Commercial oats in gluten-free diet: A persistent risk for celiac patients. Front Nutr. 2022;9:1-6.

61. Cohen IS, Day AS, Shaoul R. Gluten in celiac disease-more or less? Rambam Maimonides Med J. 2019;10(1):1-6.

62. Zysk W, Glabska D, Guzek D. Role of front-of-package gluten-free product labeling in a pair-matched study in women with and without celiac disease on a gluten-free diet. Nutrients. 2019;11(2):1-14.

63. De magistris T, Belarbi H, Hellali W. Examining non-celiac consumers of gluten-free products: an empirical evidence in Spain. In: Rodrigo L, editor. Celiac disease and non-celiac gluten sensitivity. London: IntechOpen; 2017. p. 1-14.

64. Wieser H, Segura V, Ruiz-Carnicer Á, Sousa C, Comino I. Food safety and cross-contamination of gluten-free products: a narrative review. Nutrients. 2021;13(7):1-14.

65. Colombo F, Di Lorenzo C, Biella S, Bani C, Restani P. Ancient and modern cereals as ingredients of the gluten-free diet: are they safe enough for celiac consumers? Foods. 2021;10(4):1-21.

66. Paveley WF. From aretaeus to crosby: a history of coeliac disease. BMJ. 1988;297:**1646-9**.

67. Cataldo F, Montalto G. Celiac disease in the developing countries: A new and challenging public health problem. World J Gastroenterol. 2007;13(15):**2153-9**.

68. Makovicky P, Makovicky P, Caja F, Rimarova K, Samasca G, Vannucci L. Celiac disease and gluten-free diet: past, present, and future. Gastroenterol Hepatol Bed Bench. 2020;13(1):**1-7**.

69. Soliman A, Laham M, Jour C, Shaat M, Souikey F, Itani M, et al. Linear growth of children with celiac disease after the first two years on glutenfree diet:

a controlled study. Acta Bio Medica Atenei Parm. 2019;90:**20-7**.

70. Bascuñán KA, Elli L, Vecchi M, Scricciolo A, Mascaretti F, Parisi M, et al. Mediterranean gluten-free diet: is it a fair bet for the treatment of gluten- related disorders? Front Nutr. 2020;7:1-8.

71. Aljada B, Zohni A, El-Matary W. The gluten-free diet for celiac disease and beyond. Nutrients. 2021;13(11):1-22.

72. Lerner BA, Phan LT, Yates S, Rundle AG, Green PH, Lebwohl B. Detection of gluten in gluten-free labeled restaurant food: analysis of crowd-sourced data. Am J Gastroenterol. 2019;114(5):**792-7**.

73. Raehsler SL, Choung RS, Marietta EV, Murray JA. Accumulation of heavy metals in people on a gluten-free diet. Clin Gastroenterol Hepatol. 2018;16(2):**244-51**.

74. Mancuso C, Barisani D. Food additives can act as triggering factors in celiac disease: Current knowledge based on a critical review of the literature. World J Clin Cases. 2019;7(8):**917-27**.

75. Cardo A, Churruca I, Lasa A, Navarro V, Vázquez-Polo M, Perez-Junkera G, et al. Nutritional imbalances in adult celiac patients following a gluten-free diet. Nutrients. 2021;13(8):1-18.

76. Demirkesen I, Ozkaya B. Recent strategies for tackling the problems in gluten-free diet and products. Crit Rev Food Sci Nutr. 2022;62(3):**571-97**.

77. Kreutz JM, Adriaanse MP, Van der Ploeg EM, Vreugdenhil AC. Narrative review: nutrient deficiencies in adults and children with treated and untreated celiac disease. Nutrients. 2020;12(2):1-23.

78. Lerner A, O'Bryan T, Matthias T. Navigating the gluten-free boom: the dark side of gluten free diet. Front Pediatr. 2019;7:1-8.

79. Martínez-Martinez MI, Alegre-Martínez A, García-Ibánez J, Cauli O. Quality of life in people with coeliac disease: psychological and socioeconomic aspects. Endocr Metab Immune Disord Drug Targets. 2019;19(2):**116-20**.

80. Penny HA, Baggus EM, Rej A, Snowden JA, Sanders DS. Non-responsive coeliac disease: a comprehensive review from the NHS england national centre for refractory coeliac disease. Nutrients. 2020;12(1):1-15.

81. Gladys K, Dardzrnska J, Guzek M, Adrych K, Kochan Z, Malgorzewicz S. Expanded role of a dietitian in monitoring a gluten-free diet in patients with celiac disease: implications for clinical practice. Nutrients. 2021;13(6):1- 13.

82. Paganizza S, Zanotti R, DOdorico A, Scapolo P, Canova C. Is adherence to a gluten-free diet by adult patients with celiac disease influenced by their knowledge of the gluten content of foods? Gastroenterol Nurs. 2019;42(1):**55-64**.

83. Jamieson JA, Gougeon L. Adults following a gluten-free diet report little

dietary guidance in a pilot survey exploring relationships between dietary knowledge, management, and adherence in Nova Scotia, Canada. Nutr Res. 2019;66:**107-14**.

84. Connan V, Marcon MA, Mahmud FH, Assor E, Martincevic I, Bandsma RH, et al. Online education for gluten-free diet teaching: Development and usability testing of an e-learning module for children with concurrent celiac disease and type 1 diabetes. Pediatr Diabetes. 2019;20(3):**293-303**.

85. Caio G, Ciccocioppo R, Zoli G, De Giorgio R, Volta U. Therapeutic options for coeliac disease: What else beyond gluten-free diet? Dig Liver Dis. 2020;52(2):**130-7**.

86. Al Ibrahmi B, Bour A. A short update on new approaches to celiac disease. Acta Biomed Atenei Parm. 2022;93(6):1-8.

87. Machado MV. New developments in celiac disease treatment. Int J Mol Sci. 2023;24(2):1-17.

88. García-Molina MD, Giménez MJ, Sánchez-León S, Barro F. Gluten free wheat: are we there? Nutrients. 2019;11(3):1-17.

89. Guzmán-López MH, Sánchez-León S, Marín-Sanz M, Comino I, Segura V, Vaquero L, et al. Oral consumption of bread from an RNAi wheat line with strongly silenced gliadins elicits no immunogenic response in a pilot study with celiac disease patients. Nutrients. 2021;13(12):1-13.

90. Yoosuf S, Makharia GK. Evolving therapy for celiac disease. Front Pediatr. 2019;7:1-18.

91. Graça C, Lima A, Raymundo A, Sousa I. Sourdough fermentation as a tool to improve the nutritional and health-promoting properties of its derived-products. Fermentation. 2021;7(4):1-17.

92. Heredia-Sandoval NG, Calderón de la Barca AM, Carvajal-Millán E, Islas-Rubio AR. Amaranth addition to enzymatically modified wheat flour improves dough functionality, bread immunoreactivity and quality. Food Funct. 2018;9(1):**534-40**.

93. Lamacchia C, Landriscina L, D'Agnello P. Changes in wheat kernel proteins induced by microwave treatment. Food Chem. 2016;197:**634-40**.

94. Gazikalovic I, Mijalkovic J, Sekuljica N, Jakovetic Tanaskovic S, Dukic Vukovic A, Mojovic L, et al. Synergistic effect of enzyme hydrolysis and microwave reactor pretreatment as an efficient procedure for gluten content reduction. Foods. 2021;10(9):1-23.

95. Alhassan E, Yadav A, Kelly CP, Mukherjee R. Novel nondietary therapies for celiac disease. Cell Mol Gastroenterol Hepatol. 2019;8(3):**335-45**.

96. Tye-Din JA, Anderson RP, Ffrench RA, Brown GJ, Hodsman P, Siegel M, et al. The effects of ALV003 pre-digestion of gluten on immune response and

symptoms in celiac disease in vivo. Clin Immunol. 2010;134(3):289- 95.

97. Lähdeaho ML, Kaukinen K, Laurila K, Vuotikka P, Koivurova OP, Kärjä-Lahdensuu T, et al. Glutenase ALV003 attenuates gluten-induced mucosal injury in patients with celiac disease. Gastroenterology. 2014;146(7):1649- 58.

98. Murray JA, Kelly CP, Green PH, Marcantonio A, Wu TT, Mäki M, et al. No difference between latiglutenase and placebo in reducing villous atrophy or improving symptoms in patients with symptomatic celiac disease. Gastroenterology. 2017;152(4):787-98.

99. Syage JA, Murray JA, Green PH, Khosla C. Latiglutenase improves symptoms in seropositive celiac disease patients while on a gluten-free diet. Dig Dis Sci. 2017;62(9):**2428-32**.

100. Murray JA, Syage JA, Wu TT, Dickason MA, Ramos AG, Van Dyke C, et al. Latiglutenase protects the mucosa and attenuates symptom severity in patients with celiac disease exposed to a gluten challenge. Gastroenterology. 2022;163(6):1510-21.

101. National library of medicine. Prospective, Randomized, double-blind, placebo-controlled, crossover study of the efficacy and safety of latiglutenase treatment in symptomatic celiac disease patients maintained on a gluten-free diet while undergoing periodic gluten exposure [Online]. 2023 [Accessed 16 August 2023]. Available from: https://clinicaltrials.gov/study/NCT04243551

102. Pultz IS, Hill M, Vitanza JM, Wolf C, Saaby L, Liu T, et al. Gluten degradation, pharmacokinetics, safety, and tolerability of tak-062, an engineered enzyme to treat celiac disease. Gastroenterology. 2021;161(1):81-93.

103. Tack GJ, van de Water JM, Bruins MJ, Kooy-Winkelaar EM, van Bergen J, Bonnet P, et al. Consumption of gluten with gluten-degrading enzyme by celiac patients: a pilot-study. World J Gastroenterol. 2013;19(35):**5837-47**.

104. Smecuol E. Effect of the endopeptidase AN-PEP on gluten exposure in real life in celiac disease patients treated with a long-term gluten-free diet. exploratory, interventional, prospective, controlled and double blind study [Online]. 2023 [Accessed 16 August 2023]. Available at: https://clinicaltrials.gov/study/NCT04788797

105. Pultz IS, Hill M, Vitanza JM, Wolf C, Saaby L, Liu T, et al. Gluten degradation, pharmacokinetics, safety, and tolerability of tak-062, an engineered enzyme to treat celiac disease. Gastroenterology. 2021;161(1):81-93.

106. Sample DA, Sunwoo HH, Huynh HQ, Rylance HL, Robert CL, Xu BW, et al. AGY, a Novel egg yolk-derived anti-gliadin antibody, is safe for patients with celiac disease. Dig Dis Sci. 2017;62(5):**1277-85**.

107. National library of medicine. A randomized, double-blind, placebo controlled, crossover trial to evaluate safety and efficacy of AGY in persons

with celiac disease age > 10 years [Online]. 2019 [Accessed 16 August 2023]. Available from: https://clinicaltrials.gov/study/NCT03707730

108. National library of medicine. A two-part, randomized, double-blind, placebo-controlled study to evaluate the safety and systemic exposure of single escalating administrations and repeated administration of BL-7010 in well-controlled celiac patients [Online]. 2017 [Accessed 16 August 2023]. Available from: https://clinicaltrials.gov/study/NCT01990885

109. Paterson BM, Lammers KM, Arrieta MC, Fasano A, Meddings JB. The safety, tolerance, pharmacokinetic and pharmacodynamic effects of single doses of AT-1001 in coeliac disease subjects: a proof of concept study. Aliment Pharmacol Ther. 2007;26(5):**757-66**.

110. Leffler DA, Kelly CP, Abdallah HZ, Colatrella AM, Harris LA, Leon F, et al. A randomized, double-blind study of larazotide acetate to prevent the activation of celiac disease during gluten challenge. Am J Gastroenterol. 2012;107(10):1-9.

111. Kelly CP, Green PH, Murray JA, DiMarino A, Colatrella A, Leffler DA, et al. Larazotide acetate in patients with coeliac disease undergoing a gluten challenge: a randomised placebo-controlled study. Aliment Pharmacol Ther. 2013;37(2):**252-62**.

112. Chibbar R, Dieleman LA. The gut microbiota in celiac disease and probiotics. Nutrients. 2019;11(10):1-18.

113. Martinello F, Roman CF, Souza PA. Effects of probiotic intake on intestinal bifidobacteria of celiac patients. Arq Gastroenterol. 2017;54(2):**85-90**.

114. Ali B, Khan AR. Efficacy of probiotics in management of celiac disease. Cureus. 2022;14(2):e22031.

115. National library of medicine. Exploratory, randomized, double-blind, placebo-controlled study on the effects of bifidobacterium infantis in active celiac disease [Online]. 2012 [Accessed 16 August 2023]. Available at: https://clinicaltrials.gov/study/NCT01257620

116. Büchold C, Hils M, Gerlach U, Weber J, Pelzer C, Heil A, et al. Features of ZED1227: the first-in-class tissue transglutaminase inhibitor undergoing clinical evaluation for the treatment of celiac disease. Cells. 2022;11(10):1- 20.

117. Schuppan D, Mäki M, Lundin KE, Isola J, Friesing-Sosnik T, Taavela J, et al. A randomized trial of a transglutaminase 2 inhibitor for celiac disease. N Engl J Med. 2021;385(1):**35-45**.

118. Cerf-Bensussan N, Schuppan D. The promise of novel therapies to abolish gluten immunogenicity in celiac disease. Gastroenterology. 2021;161(1):21-4.

119. Sandborn WJ, Mattheakis LC, Modi NB, Pugatch D, Bressler B, Lee S, et al. PTG-100, an Oral α4β7 antagonist peptide: preclinical development and

phase 1 and 2a studies in ulcerative colitis. Gastroenterology. 2021;161(6):1853-64.

120. National library of medicine. A phase 1b study of PTG-100 in patients with celiac disease [Online]. 2022 [Accessed 16 August 2023]. Available from: https://clinicaltrials.gov/study/NCT04524221

121. National library of medicine. Vedolizumab induction may prevent celiac enteritis after gluten challenge in established celiac patients in histological remission [Online]. 2018 [Accessed 16 August 2023]. Available from: https://clinicaltrials.gov/study/NCT02929316

122. National library of medicine. A phase II study of CCX282-B in patients with celiac disease [Online]. 2023 [Accessed 20 August 2023]. Available from: https://clinicaltrials.gov/ct2/show/NCT00540657

123. Kivelä L, Caminero A, Leffler DA, Pinto-Sanchez MI, Tye-Din JA, Lindfors K. Current and emerging therapies for coeliac disease. Nat Rev Gastroenterol Hepatol. 2021;18(3):**181-95**.

124. Cellier C, Bouma G, van Gils T, Khater S, Malamut G, Crespo L, et al. Safety and efficacy of AMG 714 in patients with type 2 refractory coeliac disease: a phase 2a, randomised, double-blind, placebo-controlled, parallel-group study. Lancet Gastroenterol Hepatol. 2019;4(12):**960-70**.

125. Lähdeaho ML, Scheinin M, Vuotikka P, Taavela J, Popp A, Laukkarinen J, et al. Safety and efficacy of AMG 714 in adults with coeliac disease exposed to gluten challenge: a phase 2a, randomised, double-blind, placebo-controlled study. Lancet Gastroenterol Hepatol. 2019;4(12):948- 59.

126. Yokoyama S, Perera PY, Waldmann TA, Hiroi T, Perera LP. Tofacitinib, a janus kinase inhibitor demonstrates efficacy in an IL-15 transgenic mouse model that recapitulates pathologic manifestations of celiac disease. J Clin Immunol. 2013;33(3):**586-94**.

127. Wauters L, Vanuytsel T, Hiele M. Celiac disease remission with tofacitinib: a case report. Ann Intern Med. 2020;173(7):585.

128. Grewal JK, Kassardjian A, Weiss GA. Successful novel use of tofacitinib for type II refractory coeliac disease. BMJ Case Rep. 2022;15(4):e244692.

129. Lähdeaho ML, Scheinin M, Vuotikka P, Taavela J, Popp A, Laukkarinen J, et al. Safety and efficacy of AMG 714 in adults with coeliac disease exposed to gluten challenge: a phase 2a, randomised, double-blind, placebo-controlled study. Lancet Gastroenterol Hepatol. 2019;4(12):948- 59.

130. Cellier C, Bouma G, van Gils T, Khater S, Malamut G, Crespo L, et al. Safety and efficacy of AMG 714 in patients with type 2 refractory coeliac disease: a phase 2a, randomised, double-blind, placebo-controlled, parallel-group study. Lancet Gastroenterol Hepatol. 2019;4(12):**960-70**.

131. National library of medicine. A phase 2b, randomized, double-blind, placebo-controlled, parallel-group study to evaluate the efficacy and safety of PRV-015 in adult patients with non-responsive celiac disease as an adjunct to a gluten-free diet [Online]. 2023 [Accessed 16 August 2023]. Available from: https://clinicaltrials.gov/study/NCT04424927

132. National Cancer Institute (NCI). Phase I study of the humanized mik-beta- 1 monoclonal antibody directed toward IL-2/IL-15R beta (CD122) that blocks IL-15 action in patients with refractory celiac disease [Online]. 2020 [Accessed 16 August 2023]. Available at: https://clinicaltrials.gov/study/NCT01893775

133. Clinical trials register. Clinical trials [Online]. 2023 [Accessed on 21 August 2023]. Available from: https://www.clinicaltrialsregister.eu/ctr-search/trial/2018-001678-10/NL#A

134. Newnham ED, Clayton-Chubb D, Nagarethinam M, Hosking P, Gibson PR. Randomised clinical trial: adjunctive induction therapy with oral effervescent budesonide in newly diagnosed coeliac disease. Aliment Pharmacol Ther. 2021;54(4):**419-28**.

135. Kelly CP, Murray JA, Leffler DA, Getts DR, Bledsoe AC, Smithson G, et al. TAK-101 nanoparticles induce gluten-specific tolerance in celiac disease: a randomized, double-blind, placebo-controlled study. gastroenterology. 2021;161(1):66-80.

136. National library of medicine. A phase 1 study of the safety and tolerability of single and multiple doses of KAN-101 in patients with celiac disease (ACeD) [Online]. 2021 [Accessed 16 August 2023]. Available at: https://clinicaltrials.gov/study/NCT04248855

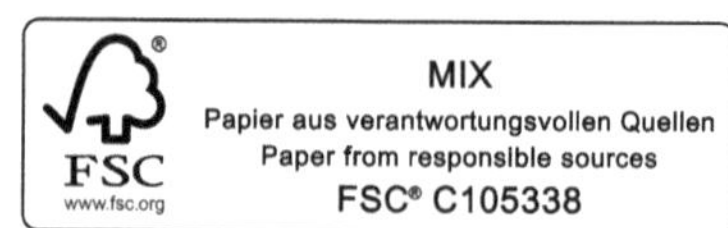

Printed by Books on Demand GmbH, Norderstedt / Germany